Department of Veterans Affairs
Health Services Research & Development Service

Evidence-based Synthesis Program

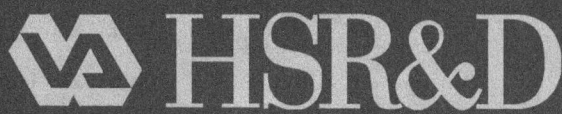

I0470879

The Assessment and Treatment of Individuals with History of Traumatic Brain Injury and Post-Traumatic Stress Disorder:
A Systematic Review of the Evidence

August 2009

Prepared for:

Department of Veterans Affairs
Veterans Health Administration
Health Services Research & Development Service
Washington, DC 20420

Prepared by:

Minneapolis Veterans Affairs Medical Center
Minnesota Evidence Synthesis Program
Center for Chronic Disease Outcomes Research
Minneapolis, MN

Investigators:

Principal Investigator
Kathleen Carlson, PhD

Co-Investigators

Shannon Kehle, PhD
Laura Meis, PhD

Research Associates

Nancy Greer, PhD
Rod MacDonald, MS
Indulis Rutks, BA

Director

Timothy J. Wilt, MD, MPH

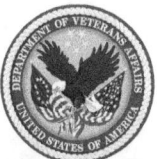

PREFACE

VA's Health Services Research and Development (HSR&D) Service works to improve the cost, quality, and outcomes of healthcare for our nation's veterans. Collaborating with VA leaders, managers, and policy makers, HSR&D focuses on important healthcare topics that are likely to have significant impact on quality improvement efforts. One significant collaborative effort is HSR&D's Evidence-based Synthesis Program (ESP). Through this program, HSR&D provides timely and accurate evidence syntheses on targeted healthcare topics. These products will be disseminated broadly throughout VA and will: inform VA clinical policy, develop clinical practice guidelines, set directions for future research to address gaps in knowledge, identify the evidence to support VA performance measures, and rationalize drug formulary decisions.

HSR&D provides funding for four ESP Centers. Each Center has an active and publicly acknowledged VA affiliation and also serves as an Evidence Based Practice Center (EPC) supported by the Agency for Healthcare Research and Quality (AHRQ). The Centers will each generate three evidence syntheses annually on clinical practice topics of key importance to VHA leadership and policymakers. A planning committee with representation from HSR&D, Patient Care Services (PCS), Quality Enhancement Research Initiative (QUERI), Office of Quality and Performance (OQP), and the VISN Clinical and Quality Management Officers, has been established to identify priority topics and key stakeholder concerns and to ensure the quality of final reports. Comments on this evidence report are welcome and can be sent to Susan Schiffner, ESP Program Manager, at Susan.Schiffner@va.gov.

This report is based on research conducted by the Minneapolis Veterans Affairs Medical Center, Minnesota Evidence Synthesis Program, and the Center for Chronic Disease Outcomes Reasearch under contract to the Department of Veterans Affairs. The findings and conclusions in this document are those of the author(s) who are responsible for its contents; the findings and conclusions do not necessarily represent the views of the Department of Veterans Affairs. Therefore, no statement in this article should be construed as an official position of the Department of Veterans Affairs.

This report is intended as a reference and not as a substitute for clinical judgment.

This report may be used, in whole or in part, as the basis for development of clinical practice guidelines and other quality enhancement tools, or as a basis for reimbursement and coverage policies. The Department of Veterans Affairs endorsement of such derivative products may not be stated or implied.

TABLE OF CONTENTS

TABLES

FIGURES

APPENDICES

EXECUTIVE SUMMARY

BACKGROUND

United States (U.S.) Veterans Affairs (VA) and Department of Defense (DoD) healthcare facilities are increasingly serving a large population of Operation Enduring Freedom and Operation Iraqi Freedom (OEF/OIF) veterans who have sustained traumatic brain injury (TBI), suffer from post-traumatic stress disorder (PTSD), or have both a history of TBI and current PTSD (TBI/PTSD). Mild TBI (mTBI) is considered the most common form of TBI. Uncertainty exists regarding the long-term health outcomes of mTBI as well as the validity of criteria used to assess for a history of this injury. Symptoms that may be attributable to mTBI are similar to symptoms of PTSD. It is unknown whether findings from civilian populations with both a history of mTBI and PTSD (mTBI/PTSD) are applicable to individuals with combat-related mTBI/PTSD. Current evidence-based practices to screen, diagnose, prospectively evaluate, and treat mTBI symptoms or PTSD may be less accurate or effective if and when these conditions co-occur. Thus, there is a need to develop an evidence base to identify best practices to define, diagnose, evaluate, and manage patients with mTBI/PTSD, particularly in U.S. veterans of OEF/OIF. We conducted a systematic literature review to address the following key questions:

1) What is the prevalence of comorbid TBI and PTSD? Does the reported prevalence vary by study population, trauma etiology, TBI severity (mild versus moderate and severe), or methods of case ascertainment?

2a) What is the relative accuracy of diagnostic tests used for assessing mTBI when mTBI is comorbid with PTSD?

2b) What is the relative accuracy of diagnostic tests used for assessing PTSD when PTSD is comorbid with mTBI?

3a) Are there psychosocial or pharmacological therapies used for treatment of mTBI and PTSD simultaneously?

3b) Are therapies for treatment of mTBI effective when mTBI is comorbid with PTSD? Is there evidence of harms?

3c) Are therapies for treatment of PTSD effective when PTSD is comorbid with mTBI? Is there evidence of harms?

This review was conducted as part of the VA Evidence Synthesis Program (ESP). The topic was nominated by the Minneapolis VA Evidence Synthesis Program Center. The report was intended to serve as an evidence-base to guide recommendations of a June 2009 VA Consensus Conference on the Diagnosis and Management of mTBI, PTSD, and pain as well as to inform healthcare practice and policy within the VA. Our key questions, scope, and work plan were refined in collaboration with a Technical Advisory Panel comprised of clinical, research, and health policy experts in TBI and PTSD.

METHODS

Literature Search

We searched the PubMed, PsycINFO, and REHABDATA databases to identify peer reviewed articles published in text journals between 1980 and June, 2009 that included patients with both a history of TBI and PTSD. Titles, abstracts, and articles were reviewed and data were extracted by investigators with knowledge of the subject area and trained in critical analysis of the literature. We attempted to assess the prevalence of TBI/PTSD in predefined patient subgroups and, for mTBI/PTSD, evaluate the quality, applicability, and strength of diagnostic accuracy studies focusing on relevance to U.S. OEF/OIF veterans using STARD and QUADAS checklists. We evaluated results from intervention trials using modifications of GRADE criteria.

Active Research

We contacted investigators of currently funded research, representatives from related VA workgroups, and authors of recently published relevant studies to collect information about ongoing research pertinent to each key question.

RESULTS

We screened 1107 references and performed a detailed full text review of 358. From these, 31 unique studies (37 references) met inclusion criteria. We also included a large telephone survey of a national sample of OEF/OIF veterans conducted by the RAND Corporation and published after peer review on their website. We excluded studies if they focused on subjects less than age 18 years of age, did not enroll individuals with probable TBI history or probable PTSD, or did not present results in a manner that addressed the key questions. The primary findings are described below.

Key Question #1

In addition to the RAND survey, 31 unique observational studies met inclusion criteria and reported prevalence of TBI/PTSD. Sample sizes ranged from 10 to 2525, though only five enrolled 200 or more subjects. No studies were U.S. population-based, though several reports focused on U.S. veterans of OEF/OIF, a key population for this report. The two largest published studies and the RAND report each evaluated approximately 2000 U.S. soldiers and veterans of OEF/OIF. Twenty-one published studies enrolled subjects with a history of mTBI (eight exclusively, including the two large studies that included U.S. veterans); the remaining described moderate and severe TBI or did not report TBI severity. Studies varied widely in their design, construction of the cohort, timing and method of case ascertainment, and definition of disease/ injury. Many studies did not report patient demographic characteristics, trauma types, or frequency of pain or mental health disorders other than PTSD. When these descriptive details were included, there was considerable variation across studies but prevalence of TBI/PTSD was generally not stratified by these potentially important variables. These factors made it impossible to pool results and greatly weakened the strength of the evidence.

Mean age of subjects ranged from 25 to 52 years and proportion female from 0% to 83%. The percent of individuals of white race ranged from 16% to 92% in the seven studies reporting race/ethnicity data. Of the 1,965 individuals included in the RAND survey, 88% were men, 66% were white (22% black), and the median age was 30 years. "Combat" (blast and non-blast) injuries accounted for most of the trauma in the eight studies involving U.S. military personnel and veterans. This was true of the RAND study as well, which was conducted with a large population of individuals previously deployed as part of OEF/OIF. Among the remaining studies involving non-veteran civilians, motor vehicle crashes were the most frequent sources of trauma.

The majority of included studies had highly selected study populations (e.g., 18 of 31 studies were based on samples in which all participants had a history of TBI and another was based on a group of patients with PTSD). Across studies, there was wide variation in the prevalence of TBI/PTSD by study population (for example, from 0% among medical patients recruited from a single-center Neurology Department to 70% in a clinical sample of patients with obsessive-compulsive disorder); trauma types (32% to 66% of participants with combat-related TBI); TBI severity (0% to 89% among individuals with mTBI and 0% to 19% among those with severe TBI); and methods of case ascertainment (5% to 66% among participants responding to self-report inventories of PTSD symptoms and 8% to 70% among those assessed through structured clinical interviews). In the RAND cohort, the prevalence levels of probable TBI history and PTSD were 19.5% and 13.8%, respectively; the prevalence of probable TBI/PTSD was 6.6%.

Key Question #2

There were no published studies addressing the relative accuracy of diagnostic tests used for assessing history or symptoms of mTBI or PTSD when one condition co-occurs with the other.

Key Question #3

There were no published studies that evaluated the effectiveness and harms of treatments for co-management of mTBI/PTSD. There were no studies that examined effectiveness of treatments specifically for PTSD or mTBI symptoms in individuals with both conditions.

Active Research:

Responses were received from 30 individuals. We identified four ongoing studies that will report prevalence of TBI/PTSD, five studies on assessment of mTBI/PTSD, three studies that address both prevalence and assessment of mTBI/PTSD, and six studies on treatment of mTBI/PTSD. One of the treatment studies identified is a randomized, controlled trial.

FUTURE RESEARCH NEEDS

Long-term prospective observational studies are needed that use standardized validated measures of both history and symptoms of TBI and PTSD to determine prevalence, severity, and long-term outcomes of TBI/PTSD, especially in veterans with history and symptoms of mTBI. Among military personnel, pre-deployment as well as post-deployment assessment should be completed using objective measures that limit ascertainment, recall, or reporting bias. Outcomes data should be stratified by clinically relevant patient characteristics, trauma etiology and severity, and time from trauma. Diagnostic accuracy studies are needed that utilize established quality methods. Randomized controlled treatment trials in populations of interest are required to evaluate the effectiveness and harms of potential therapeutic options, especially among individuals with mTBI history.

CONCLUSIONS

Reported prevalence of TBI/PTSD varies widely, likely depending on patient characteristics, trauma etiology and severity, and the disease/injury definition used and time and method of ascertainment. There is no information on the relative diagnostic accuracy of commonly used tests to assess history and symptoms of mTBI or PTSD when the conditions are co-occurring, though the prevalence of co-occurrence is likely to depend most closely on diagnostic methods, definitions, and timing of ascertainment. There is no information on the effectiveness and harms of therapies in adults with mTBI/PTSD. The reported active research studies are inadequate to address key questions 2 and 3 assessed in this review.

INTRODUCTION

Traumatic brain injury (TBI) has been defined as trauma to the head that results in a decreased level of consciousness, amnesia, other neurologic or neuropsychologic abnormalities, skull fractures, intracranial lesions, or death.[1] TBI can be caused by penetrating trauma or by blunt force, including acceleration/deceleration forces that cause the brain to collide with the skull.[1] Blunt force TBI is typically classified by level of severity, most commonly differentiated as mild, moderate, or severe. The vast majority of civilian patients that are hospitalized for TBI are diagnosed with mild TBI (mTBI).[2] While a similar ratio specific to soldiers or veterans is not readily available, mTBI is also prevalent in this population.[3] Personnel engaged in the current military operations, Operation Enduring Freedom and Operation Iraqi Freedom (OEF/OIF), are sustaining mTBI at unprecedented rates.[4] One commonly referenced report estimated that nearly 20%, or 300,000, OEF/OIF veterans had sustained a TBI during deployment,[5] many of these being mTBI. There has been much political and media interest in the rates of mTBI associated with the current conflicts. While most of those who sustain mTBI do not experience ongoing symptoms, a minority of individuals will experience some psychosocial, mental, and/or physical health problems.[6,7] Thus, there is major concern across veteran healthcare providers, particularly the U.S. Department of Veterans Affairs (VA) and Department of Defense (DoD), regarding the identification and care of mTBI.

Post-traumatic stress disorder (PTSD) is a highly prevalent and pernicious mental health problem with significant costs to the individual and society. It is an anxiety disorder characterized by avoidance behaviors, physiological hyperarousal, and re-experiencing symptoms following exposure to a traumatic event.[8] Population-based epidemiologic studies have shown that nearly 56% of people will experience a psychologically traumatic event, and between 8-12% of individuals will meet criteria for PTSD during their lifetimes.[9,10] United States (U.S.) military veterans' risk of developing PTSD is higher than the risk in the general U.S. population. The lifetime prevalence of PTSD among Vietnam veterans is estimated to be 19%.[11] Similar patterns are being observed among OEF/OIF soldiers and veterans. A study by Hoge and colleagues found that exposure to traumatic events was extremely high among OIF soldiers and Marines, with 93% to 97% having been shot at and approximately 95% having seen human remains.[12] Screening data from OIF soldiers suggest that approximately 17% of active duty soldiers and 25% of reserve soldiers may meet criteria for PTSD three to six months post-deployment.[13] Studies have found that veterans with PTSD have significant impairments in social and occupational functioning and quality of life.[14-18]

VA and DoD healthcare providers are now facing a large population of OEF/OIF veterans who have sustained TBI, particularly mTBI, and also suffer from PTSD.[19] However, the long-term health outcomes of individuals who have received diagnoses of both TBI and PTSD (TBI/PTSD), especially mTBI and PTSD (mTBI/PTSD), are poorly understood. There is concern that current evidence-based practices to define, identify, and treat mTBI and PTSD may be less accurate and/or effective when the conditions co-occur. Thus, there is a need to develop an evidence base and identify best practices for patients with this co-diagnosis. The objective of this evidence synthesis report was to systematically review and summarize the published literature that addresses the epidemiology, assessment, and treatment of adults with mTBI/PTSD.

While the epidemiologic review compares prevalence estimates of PTSD across all TBI severity levels, so as to examine any potential differences in prevalence by TBI severity, the assessment and treatment sections of this report were focused on mTBI because of the growing concerns related to this injury in the U.S. military population. We emphasized results most relevant to U.S. military personnel and veterans.

BACKGROUND

Because of the dramatic rise in the number of veterans who have sustained TBI and psychological trauma, there has been a recent spike in the literature pertaining to the overlap between the two conditions. There has been scientific debate about whether or not the history of TBI may preclude the development of PTSD.[20,21] This debate stemmed mainly from the fact that PTSD by definition involves re-experiencing of traumatic events, while TBI frequently involves amnesia for the traumatic event and, thus, no memories to re-experience. For example, a study by Sbordone and Liter found that all PTSD patients were able to provide a highly detailed recollection of events occurring within 15 minutes of the traumatic event, compared with none of the patients who had sustained TBI.[21] These authors suggested that history of TBI and development of PTSD are mutually exclusive events. However, since the time of their report, there has been continued documentation of PTSD developing in individuals with history of TBI, and co-occurring TBI/PTSD symptoms, across a variety of populations and TBI severity levels.[24-26] Thus, it is generally accepted that the two conditions can and do co-occur.

More recently, however, researchers have proposed that symptoms often attributed to mTBI could instead be due to PTSD and other mental health problems.[22,23] Hoge et al. found that, after statistical adjustment for PTSD and depression, soldiers' mTBI history (assessed three to four months after return from deployment) no longer had a statistically significant association with physical health symptoms with the exception of headaches.[22] The results of this study may reflect the normal healing process generally experienced after mTBI. It is estimated that approximately 90% of mTBI cases follow a predictable course of recovery and do not experience long-term residual symptoms requiring treatment.[6,7] A small minority of individuals may experience ongoing mTBI-related psychosocial, mental, and/or physical health problems; however, a 2008 Institute of Medicine (IOM) report on the long-term consequences of TBI cited insufficient evidence of associations between mTBI and neurocognitive deficits or limitations in psychosocial functioning.[24] Hoge et al. have suggested that definitions frequently used for both screening and eventual diagnosis of mTBI, especially in the presence of suspected PTSD, are methodologically inadequate, not validated, prone to bias, and potentially result in misattributing a chronic health condition to a large group of individuals.[23] They particularly draw comparisons and distinctions between mTBI versus moderate and severe TBI as noted in the table below.[23] Hoge et al. urge use of an approach that would "establish case definitions and evaluation tools that fulfill criteria for causation; have clinical validity and do not lead to misattribution; ensure that screening does not include nonspecific questions, is conducted near the time of injury, and maintains independence of variables; use communication strategies that promote expectations of recovery; apply knowledge from studies on the relationship between compensation and persistent post-concussive symptoms to ensure that disability regulations do not generate disability; … [develop and evaluate] evidence-based step-care and collaborative care models; and reduce the impact of flawed assumptions, conformity to consensus processes, and lack of scientific rigor on health policies and outcomes."[23] While the viewpoints by Hoge et al. are disputed for clinical purposes,[28] it is noteworthy that some of their suggestions, such as stricter standardization of case definitions, would result in higher quality evidence for scientific purposes, upon which practice guidelines specific to patients with mTBI/PTSD could be based.

Comparison of Mild TBI with Moderate and Severe TBI*		
Variable	**Mild TBI (Concussion)**	**Moderate and Severe TBI**
Clinical definition	Loss of consciousness lasting <30 minutes, any alteration of consciousness, or post-traumatic amnesia lasting <24 hrs; some definitions include Glasgow Coma Scale score of 13 to 15	Loss of consciousness lasting ≥ 30 minutes to prolonged coma, post-traumatic amnesia lasting ≥24 hr up to permanently, or Glasgow Coma score as low as 3
Focal neurologic signs	Usually none or transient	Frequently present
Neuroimaging with CT or MRI	Usually negative	Diagnostic
Natural History	Full recovery is usual; there is lack of consensus on the natural history of concussion and post-concussive symptoms	Natural history and recovery are directly related to the severity of the injury and functional neuroanatomy
Case definitions and specificity of injury sequelae	Case definitions of post-concussive syndrome have low reliability and validity and show poor correlation with one another; there are high rates of these symptoms in healthy populations and high rates of "post-concussion syndrome" after non-head injuries	Injury sequelae are not debated
Predictors of persistent symptoms or disability	Psychological factors (e.g., depression, anxiety, or PTSD), compensation and litigation, and negative expectations and beliefs are the strongest risk factors	Directly related to injury characteristics
Neurocognitive testing	Often inconclusive beyond the period of acute injury	Essential and valuable component of on-going clinical care
Neuronal-cell damage	Metabolic and ionic processes caused by axonal twisting or stretching; these can lead to secondary disconnection	Combination of cellular disruption directly related to injury and metabolic, vascular, and ionic processes
Epidemiologic evidence of causation between injury and sequelae	Inconsistent and debated	Not debated

*CT denotes computed tomography, MRI magnetic resonance imaging, PTSD post-traumatic stress disorder and TBI traumatic brain injury.

Note: Table adapted from Hoge et al.[23]

There seems to be little convergent data on the prevalence, health outcomes, and treatment of TBI/PTSD. Previous reviews have highlighted the widely variable rates of overlap between diagnosis of TBI and PTSD.[29-31] For example, McMillan reported that the prevalence of cases with both diagnoses ranged across studies from 1% to more than 50%,[29] while Kim et al. similarly reported a range from 3% to 59%.[30] Discrepancies in the reported epidemiology of TBI/PTSD may be due to differences in the true prevalence of these conditions specific to different types of trauma, levels of trauma severity, and/or baseline characteristics of the study population. Additionally, as indicated above, the methods of case ascertainment, that is, the methods, criteria, and cut-offs used to epidemiologically define and study TBI and/or PTSD "cases," can vary widely.[32] It is important to examine reported prevalence of TBI/PTSD across these potentially significant sub-categories (severity, etiology, study population, and case ascertainment) to gain a better understanding of the overlap between the two conditions.

Determining the etiology of presenting problems in individuals who have a history of mTBI as well as probable current PTSD may be complicated. While mTBI is considered a historical diagnosis and should not require the presence of current symptoms for a diagnosis to be assigned, this understanding may not be shared across all clinical disciplines that encounter mTBI patients. A number of symptoms and associated problems are common to both mTBI and PTSD. These symptoms include sleep disturbance, fatigue, depressed mood, concentration and memory problems, irritability, and reduced cognitive processing speed.[26] As noted by Hoge et al., PTSD and depression may be important confounders of problems seemingly associated with an mTBI event or other physical health problems.[22] Problems due to mTBI can also obstruct patients' abilities to verbalize and describe symptoms of either condition.[33] Research has also suggested that the presentation of PTSD symptoms may actually vary among individuals with and without a history of mTBI, such that different constellations of symptoms are more prominent among those with a history of brain injury (e.g., dreams, nightmares, and hyperarousal) than among those without history of brain injury (e.g., intrusive recollections).[34] Additionally, the presence of other problems that commonly occur with both conditions (e.g., alcohol use, depression) may interfere with attempts to develop and complete an accurate diagnostic profile.[33]

It remains unknown how well diagnostic instruments currently used for assessing history and symptoms of mTBI or PTSD perform in individuals with both conditions. Without this understanding, including how rates of co-occurrence vary with different approaches to assessment, conclusions regarding the true presence and extent of overlap between mTBI and PTSD cannot be reached. Additionally, as each condition could yield alternative explanations for symptomology, accurate and differential diagnosis provides important implications for treatment. For example, avoidance of previous activities can be due to either symptoms of PTSD or the development of mTBI-related cognitive deficits. Intrusive thoughts can be explained through attempts by the patient to fill memory gaps caused by mTBI or through symptoms of PTSD.[26,35] As a result, developing and evaluating appropriate treatment recommendations remains tied to accurate assessment and diagnosis of both mTBI and PTSD.

Efficacious treatment for individuals with mTBI/PTSD is of importance to VA and DoD as well as the private healthcare sector. Initial data suggest that a large number of veterans with history and/or diagnoses of both mTBI and PTSD are presenting for treatment; one study examining outcomes and service utilization of OIF veterans one-year post-deployment found that 65% of those with mTBI/PTSD reported seeking treatment for concerns related to reintegration.[19] Fortunately, there are a number of efficacious psychological and pharmacological treatments for PTSD. The treatments with the strongest evidence are cognitive-behavioral psychotherapies. Effect sizes for cognitive-behavioral treatments, such as prolonged exposure therapy and cognitive processing therapy, range from medium to very large when compared to no-treatment conditions, and from small to large when compared to other psychological or psychiatric treatments.[36] Among veterans, high quality studies have shown that 40% to 50% of patients no longer meet criteria for PTSD following either prolonged exposure or cognitive processing therapy.[37,38] Preliminary data also suggest that such therapies will be helpful for OEF/OIF veterans. A small, ongoing trial of prolonged exposure among OEF/OIF veterans has shown a 50% reduction in PTSD symptoms following treatment.[39] Data regarding the treatment of mTBI symptoms are less robust than the evidence for treatment of PTSD; however, there is evidence that providing psychoeducation regarding the typical sequelae, expected course of recovery, and compensatory strategies soon after injury may be effective in facilitating the return to premorbid functioning.[40,41] The VA and DoD have recommended early education as a treatment of choice for those with a history of mTBI.[6]

While efficacious treatments for both mTBI symptoms and PTSD exist, patients presenting with both a history of mTBI and PTSD may need unique therapies. Patients with both conditions may experience a differential response to standard treatments compared to those with only mTBI history or PTSD. Bryant and Hopwood have identified mechanisms by which mTBI symptoms may interfere with evidence-based treatments for PTSD.[20] They note that physical pain, which frequently occurs after mTBI,[42] may limit the extent to which patients can engage in empirically supported treatments that involve in-person exposure to anxiety producing situations. They additionally note that cognitive limitations may make it necessary to modify cognitive-behavioral therapies, and that emotion regulation and impulse control problems may complicate the use of exposure techniques. It is unknown whether or how PTSD may conversely interfere with treatment of patients who have developed symptoms due to mTBI.

This review seeks to summarize the literature published between 1980 and June, 2009 that is specific to the epidemiology of TBI/PTSD, and to the assessment and treatment of mTBI/PTSD. It is important to note that, consistent with its definition, we have conceptualized "TBI" as a historical event and do not require the presence of current symptoms to enumerate TBI cases. However, even though a clinical interview is necessary to render a confirmed TBI diagnosis, we have included in this evidence review studies in which survey-based screening measures were used to enumerate both "probable TBI" history and current "probable PTSD." Additionally, we have included studies that were based on data from the VA's post-deployment screening program, in which "symptomatic probable TBI" cases are identified based on historical TBI-related events plus current symptoms potentially attributable to a TBI. We have been careful to specify studies based on screening versus clinical cases when possible.

METHODS

TOPIC DEVELOPMENT

This topic was nominated by the Center for Chronic Disease Outcomes Research, Minneapolis VA Medical Center, in consultation with the Polytrauma/Blast-related Injuries QUERI and the VA Evidence Synthesis Program. The key questions and scope of this review were refined based on input from Technical Advisory Panel members Matthew Friedman, MD, Robin Hurley, MD, Nancy Bernardy, PhD, and Katherine Helmick, MS, CNRN, CRNP.

The final key questions were:

1) What is the observed prevalence of comorbid TBI and PTSD? Does the reported prevalence vary by study population, trauma etiology, TBI severity, or methods of case ascertainment?

2a) What is known about the relative accuracy of diagnostic tests used for assessing mTBI when comorbid with PTSD?

2b) What is known about the relative accuracy of diagnostic tests used for assessing PTSD when comorbid with mTBI?

3a) Are there psychosocial or pharmacological therapies used for treatment of mTBI and PTSD simultaneously?

3b) Are therapies for treatment of mTBI effective when mTBI is comorbid with PTSD? Is there evidence of harms?

3c) Are therapies for treatment of PTSD effective when PTSD is comorbid with mTBI? Is there evidence of harms?

SEARCH STRATEGY

A study search coordinator developed the search strategy with input from the principal investigators (Appendix A). We searched PubMed, PsycINFO, and REHABDATA databases for articles published from 1980 to June, 2009. The search was limited to studies involving human subjects and published in English. Reference lists from studies related to the key questions were searched for additional research studies. TBI was operationalized as a history of confusion, disorientation, or loss of consciousness resulting from a force to the head.[43] Included studies must have enrolled participants with a self-reported history of probable TBI, or diagnosed TBI history, regardless of the presence of current TBI-related symptoms. PTSD was operationalized as the development of symptoms characterized as Post-traumatic Stress Disorder by the Diagnostic and Statistical Manual (DSM-III, DSM-III-R, DSM-IV, or DSM-IV-TR).[44-47] Included studies must have had participants with DSM-III or DSM-IV diagnoses of or positive screens for PTSD as determined through semi-structured interview, clinical diagnosis of PTSD, or scores exceeding cutoffs indicating probable diagnosis of PTSD on self-report inventories.

A description of the search strategy used to identify ongoing and unpublished research studies is presented in the Active Research section below.

STUDY SELECTION

Titles and abstracts (when available) from all references identified in the literature search process were reviewed by a study investigator (KC, SK, LM). The initial screening was designed to identify peer-reviewed, English language articles published after 1980 that included an adult population with probable or diagnosed history of TBI and probable or diagnosed PSTD and were related to one or more of the key questions or that might provide background information. Studies of all design types were considered. Full-text versions of articles that potentially met these criteria were then obtained for further review. We excluded studies if they included more than 10% of subjects less than age 18 years, did not enroll individuals with a history of probable TBI or probable or diagnosed PTSD, or did not present results in a manner that addressed the key questions. Studies that did not meet inclusion criteria for key questions but were considered of special relevance because they were of high methodologic quality or provided evidence potentially, but not directly, relevant to the key questions were included as secondary results.

DATA ABSTRACTION

A content expert abstracted data onto standardized forms (Appendix B) from each article that met the study selection criteria. Results were reviewed with another member of the research team. For Key Question #1, we abstracted the study setting and overall population (e.g., military, veteran, civilian), as well as population demographics (gender, age, race/ethnicity, education level, disability seeking status, presence of pain or mental health disorders other than PTSD), trauma etiology (e.g., combat, terror, motor vehicle, assault), severity of TBI (mild, moderate, severe, and how defined), number of and time since trauma(s), and method(s) used to ascertain, define, and enumerate TBI and PTSD cases (administrative data, self-report, clinical screening, structured interview, neuropsychiatric evaluation). Numerator (TBI/PTSD) and denominator (total study population) data were collected to allow reporting of prevalence by study population. We included studies that assessed for PTSD in patients with a reported history of TBI as well as studies that assessed for both TBI and PTSD across more heterogeneous patient populations.

We attempted to address Key Question #2 using established methods as outlined by Bossuyt et al.[47] and Leeflang et al.[48] Population, trauma, and case assessment data were abstracted as defined for Key Question #1. In addition, if reported, we noted the operationalized cut-off scores for tests used to diagnose mTBI and/or PTSD (including screening instruments, clinical interviews, neuropsychological batteries), the names of diagnostic reference tests used for comparison, and the operationalized cut-off scores for these reference tests. Other data we sought to abstract included whether those administering tests for mTBI or PTSD were blinded to results of the other assessment methods, the time interval between administration of the tests, whether treatments were received between tests, and the methods used to calculate or compare the diagnostic accuracy and statistical uncertainty. We attempted to determine if comparator test findings would lead to reclassification of disease/injury presence or treatment versus the control diagnostic test. We sought to examine variability in reports of diagnostic accuracy by population subtype.

For Key Question #3, we included only studies in which at least 80% of the participants were diagnosed with both mTBI and PTSD or the outcomes were stratified for those with both diagnoses. We sought to abstract results from studies of psychological or pharmacological therapies that simultaneously targeted symptoms of mTBI and PTSD or from studies that treated only one of the conditions in individuals with both conditions. Because we expected to identify few studies that would include either a wait-list control or other comparison group, we included studies of treatment outcomes without a comparison group. The outcomes of interest were PTSD symptomology (self-report or clinician-assessed), mTBI symptomology (self-report or objective performance measures), functional status/ability, pain, and quality of life. When data were available, outcomes at baseline, post-treatment, short (one- to six-months), medium (six-months to one year), and long-term (greater than one year) follow-up were recorded. Harms that occurred due to administering a treatment designed for only one of the conditions to a participant with mTBI/PTSD were documented as were the characteristics of the study setting (e.g., veteran or community hospital).

QUALITY ASSESSMENT

We attempted to rate the quality of randomized controlled trials, cohort studies, and case-control studies as good, fair, or poor based on criteria specific to the study design type.[49] Cross-sectional studies, case series, and case reports were considered of low methodologic quality. We assessed studies for applicability to U.S. OEF/OIF veterans. Evidence tables were organized by key questions and conclusions were drawn based on qualitative syntheses of the evidence. We also sought to evaluate the overall quality of the evidence for each main outcome as proposed by the GRADE Working Group.[50]

DATA SYNTHESIS

We constructed evidence tables showing the study characteristics and results for all included studies, organized by key question, intervention, or clinical condition, as appropriate. We critically analyzed studies to compare their characteristics, methods, and findings. We compiled a summary of findings for each key question or clinical topic, and drew conclusions based on qualitative synthesis of the findings. We did not conduct pooled analyses due to marked heterogeneity in study design, cohort creation, patient demographic characteristics, trauma type, etiology, assessment methodology, and disease/injury definition. We report individual study results and summarize findings across these key variables.

ACTIVE RESEARCH

We identified ongoing and/or unpublished funded research related to the key questions by searching the VA HSR&D research database (http://www.hsrd.research.va.gov/research), the Computer Retrieval of Information on Scientific Projects (CRISP) database (http://crisp.cit. nih.gov/crisp), the Clinical Trials database (http://www.clinicaltrials.gov), the *meta*Register of Controlled Trials (http://www.controlled-trials.com/mrct), and the Department of Defense Congressionally Directed Medical Research Program (CDMRP) database. We contacted the HSR&D Program Managers for Long Term Care and Mental Health; individuals associated with the National Center for PTSD; the Physical Medicine and Rehabilitation TBI/Polytrauma Program; the Polytrauma/Blast-Related Injuries QUERI; the War Related Illness and Injury Study Center (WRIISC); and key authors in the field. Members of our Technical Advisory Panel and the Polytrauma/Blast-related Injuries QUERI provided additional contacts. Individuals were contacted once by e-mail and asked to provide a brief protocol or to complete a survey to capture information about related research projects. This survey was adapted from a survey used by the Oregon Evidence-based Practice Center in a systematic review of pain in patients with polytrauma.[51] There was no further attempt to contact individuals who did not respond to our initial e-mail request.

PEER REVIEW

A draft version of this report was sent to peer reviewers that included members of our Technical Advisory Panel; participants in the VA consensus conference on practice recommendations for treatment of veterans with mTBI, PTSD, and pain; and Dr. Charles W. Hoge, Director of the Division of Psychiatry and Neuroscience at Walter Reed Army Institute of Research. Peer reviewer comments were compiled, responses were prepared (Appendix C), and resulting edits were incorporated into the final version of this report.

RESULTS

LITERATURE FLOW

The combined library contained 1107 citations, of which we reviewed 358 articles at the full-text level. From those 358 articles, we identified 31 unique studies (described in 37 references) that addressed the key questions (Figure 1). Studies were excluded because they were published prior to 1980, included more than 10% of participants less than age 18 years, did not enroll individuals with history of probable TBI or probable PTSD, or did not present results in a manner that addressed the key questions. A study by the RAND Corporation was included under primary results (not depicted in diagram). The RAND study assessed both probable TBI history and PTSD in a large, presumably nationally-representative sample of U.S. military personnel. While it was not published in a peer-reviewed journal, the report was peer-reviewed, published by the RAND Corporation, and is available on the RAND website.[5] An additional five studies were included under secondary results (not depicted in flow diagram).

Figure 1. Published data search and selection

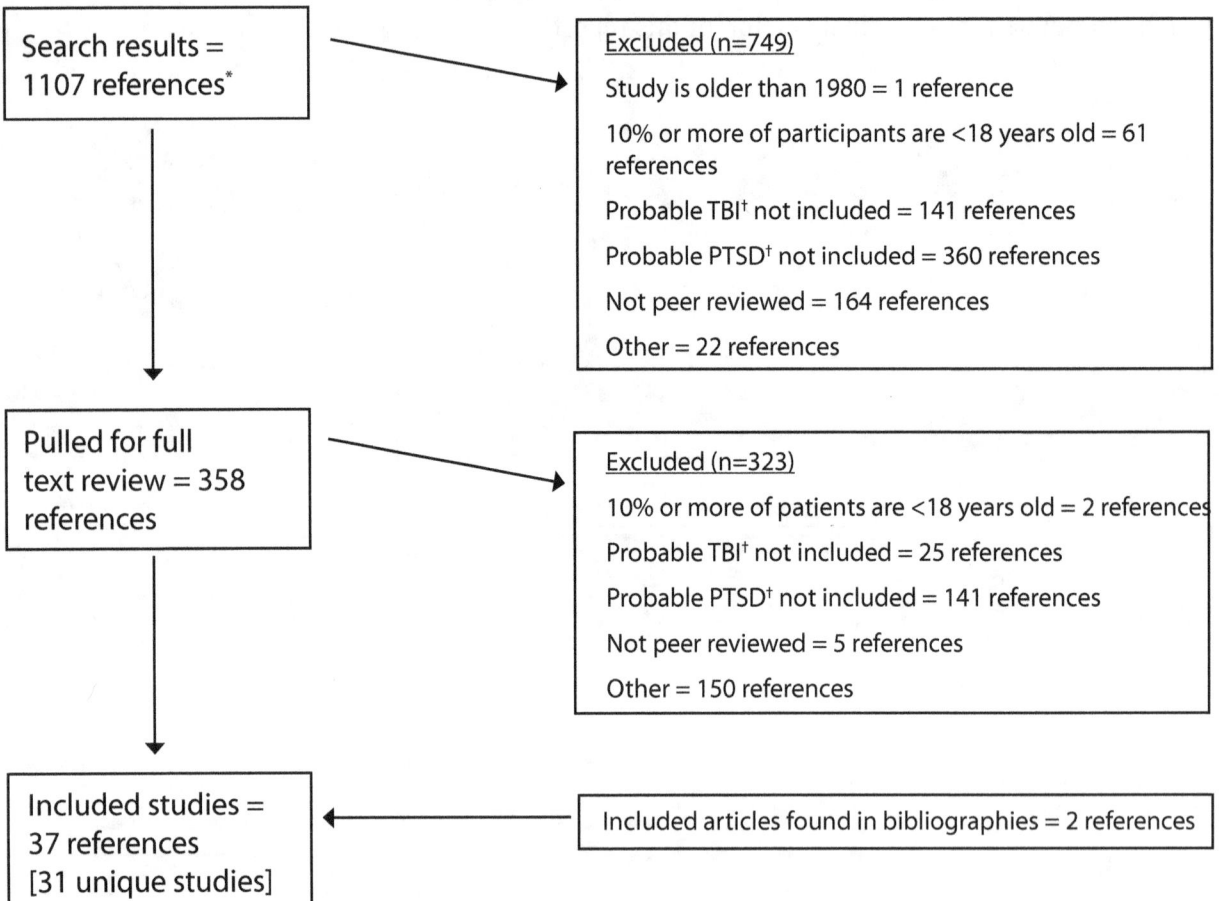

*Search results from PubMed (700), PsycInfo (552) and REHABDATA (123) were combined, removing duplicate entries (268).
† "Probable" TBI and PTSD are defined on page 6 and include positive "screens" based on self-report measures as well as clinical diagnoses.

Key Question #1.

What is the observed prevalence of comorbid TBI and PTSD? Does the reported prevalence vary by study population, trauma etiology, TBI severity, or methods of case ascertainment?

Summary of Findings

There were 31 unique studies that reported prevalence of TBI/PTSD. We also included a telephone survey of a national sample of OEF/OIF veterans conducted by the RAND Corporation that was peer reviewed and published electronically on their website yielding a total of 32 unique studies. Studies varied considerably by design, population, trauma etiology and severity, presence of pain or mental health disorders other than PTSD, methods and timing of case ascertainment, and definitions of disease/injury and severity. Additionally, while clinically relevant baseline characteristics were sometimes reported, prevalence of TBI/PTSD was rarely stratified by these variables. Therefore, results could not be pooled across studies, few patterns could be discerned, and reliable outcome estimates could not be obtained for key patient groups. A few studies uniquely enrolled or excluded subjects with a particular characteristic (e.g., men; military veterans). We attempted to separately describe findings from studies that were unique to the military or veteran population.

Study Details (Table 1; Appendix D)

Description of studies reporting prevalence of TBI/PTSD
Thirty-one unique published studies meeting inclusion criteria and enrolling between 10 and 2525 participants (majority less than 200) reported prevalence of TBI/PTSD among participants.[21,22,52-81] Additionally, the study by the RAND Corporation, which enrolled 1965 participants, reported prevalence of TBI/PTSD.[5] The two largest of the published studies and the RAND report involved U.S. military personnel.[5,22,55] A summary of characteristics across published studies is presented in Table 1. Details on study design, population characteristics, assessment methods, and prevalence data for each of the published studies and, separately, the RAND study, are tabulated in Appendix D (Tables 1 and 2).

Study design and location
Many studies were single center and nearly all assessed TBI/PTSD status in patients who had been previously hospitalized or received care in an emergency room specifically related to their trauma. Because individuals who have experienced a TBI, especially mTBI, or who have PTSD may not present to medical facilities for TBI/PTSD-related symptoms, findings from most of the identified studies may not provide accurate population estimates (even for military veterans) for the prevalence of both conditions, particularly mTBI/PTSD. One study (n=144) utilized a case-control design;[56] the remaining were mostly cohort or cross-sectional studies. One small case series enrolled ten subjects.[65] The majority of studies were conducted in the U.S. (n=16),[21,22,52-55,57,58,63,67,71-74,79,81] followed by the United Kingdom (n=6),[61,62,64,77,78,80] Australia (n=4),[59,68-70] Israel (n=3),[56,60,66] and Denmark (n=1).[76] The RAND report described a cross-sectional U.S. national telephone survey of OEF/OIF veterans.[5]

Patient demographic characteristics

Eight of the American studies and the RAND report evaluated U.S. military personnel.[5,22,52-55,73,79,81] In 24 of the 29 studies reporting gender, the majority of subjects were male (ranging from 53% to 100%). One U.S. study evaluating veterans was exclusive to males.[73] Among the 27 studies reporting mean age, ages averaged between 30 and 40 years; two studies had mean ages greater than 50 years.[73,79] Among the seven studies reporting race, most subjects were white (range 16% to 92%).[57,58,63,67,71,72,79] One study (n=200) included mostly non-white subjects (84%).[67] Most U.S. subjects had at least a high school education. The RAND study evaluated a military active duty and veteran population that was mostly male (89%), mostly white (66%), and had a median age of 30.[5]

TBI severity

Twenty-four studies[21,22,52,53,55,56-61,63,65,67-70,73,75-81] included subjects with a history of mTBI, 12 exclusively.[21,22,52,53,55,59-61,68-70,76] The percentage of subjects who experienced a moderate TBI ranged from 10% to 40% in 10 studies[56-58,65,67,73,75,78-80] and 100% in one study.[74] The percentage of subjects who experienced a severe TBI ranged from 5% to 62% in eight studies[56-58,65,78-81] and 100% in three studies.[62,64,66] Only two studies did not report levels of TBI severity.[71,72] The RAND study did not measure information pertinent to TBI severity.[5] However, by virtue of the study population, and the substantial proportion of respondents reporting they had received no medical care related to a TBI, the majority of individuals reporting a history of TBI were likely to have incurred mTBI.

TBI etiology

Injuries related to combat (blast and non-blast sources) accounted for most of the trauma in the studies of U.S. military personnel.[22,52-55,73,79,81] Combat-related trauma was reported exclusively in five of the eight U.S. studies involving soldiers and veterans.[52-54,73,81] Combat injury was noted in only one study outside the U.S., accounting for 25% of trauma cases in an Israeli study.[66] Trauma resulting in TBI due to motor vehicle crashes (MVC) was reported in 22 studies, ranging from 17% to 100% of the cases.[21,22,55,56-58,60-62,64-72,74,77,78,80] Five of the studies included only trauma due to MVCs.[61,65,69,70,72] Trauma due to assaults (range 3% to 58%) was reported in 10 studies[57,62,64,67,68,71,74,75,78,80] and trauma due to falls (range 8% to 39%) was also reported in 10 studies.[21,22,55,56,58,62,64,74,78,80] The case-control study, conducted in Israel, compared trauma due to terror (blast or gunshot) to non-terror trauma, mainly as a result of MVCs.[56] The RAND study did not precisely identify TBI etiology.[5] The survey asked respondents about TBI-related events that occurred while deployed.

Presence of pain or mental health disorders other than PTSD

Pain, including headaches, was reported in five studies (11% to 100% of participants).[22,53,68,69,76] Few studies reported the prevalence of any mental health disorders other than PTSD. Depression (or depressive symptoms) was the most commonly reported mental health condition, reported in nine studies.[22,57,63,65-67,71,75,80] Prevalence was less than 50% in most studies. One case series study involved participants (n=10) of which 90% had been diagnosed with obsessive-compulsive disorder.[65] Substance use disorder was reported in three studies, ranging from 14% to 42% of participants,[63,71,73] followed by anxiety disorders other than PTSD (9% to 60% of participants) reported in four studies,[57,63,71,80] and panic disorder (14% of participants) reported in one study.[71]

A major purpose of the RAND study was to assess the prevalence of depression in the OEF/OIF veteran population. Approximately 14% of the study population was deemed to have probable major depressive disorder.[5]

Definitions and ascertainment methods

Studies varied widely in their operational definitions of TBI and PTSD and the methods and timing of assessment. Methods of case ascertainment included medical records review, clinical interviews, varying scores on the Glasgow Coma Scale, self report of loss of consciousness and/or altered mental status, and receiving treatment for a head injury at a hospital. Several studies based case inclusion criteria on positive responses to TBI and/or PTSD screening measures. For example, a single cross-sectional administrative database study of 126 veterans (gender, race, and age not reported) used a positive screen on the VA 4-item TBI screening instrument to enroll participants.[53] In this study, the prevalence of TBI/PTSD was determined by assessing the percentage of individuals reported to have a probable history of TBI based on this instrument who also scored >50 on the self-reported Post-traumatic Stress Disorder Checklist (PCL). The RAND study similarly used screening instruments to assess history of TBI (the Brief Traumatic Brain Injury Screen [BTBIS]) and PTSD (PCL-Military Version [PCL-M]).[5] The time since trauma when assessments were conducted was frequently not reported. However, three longitudinal studies followed hospital TBI cohorts over time and assessed for PTSD at various reported time points since injury.[58,61,70]

Table 1. Summary of study characteristics for n=31 published unique studies reporting prevalence of TBI/PTSD

Characteristic	Range (# of participants, percents, or means)	# of studies reporting
Range of enrolled subjects	10 to 2525	31
Range of enrolled subjects in studies in which all subjects were U.S. veteran and/or active duty	43 to 2525	8
Mean age	25 to 52	27
Gender, female - %	0 to 83	29
Race, white - %	16 to 92	7
Race, non-white - %	6 to 84	7
Education, less than high school graduate - %*	3 to 48	4
Education, high school graduate or more - %*	34 to 85	5
Education, any college - %*	25 to 49	3
TBI severity (Studies not reporting TBI severity n=8)		
TBI, mild - %	19 to 100 (*11 studies 100%*)	21
TBI, moderate - %	10 to 100 (*1 study 100%*)	12
TBI, severe - %	17 to 100 (*3 studies 100%*)	12
Trauma etiology (Studies not reporting etiology n=4)		
Motor vehicle crashes - %	17 to 100 (*6 studies 100%*)	22
Assaults - %	3 to 58	11
Falls - %	8 to 39	11
Combat-related injuries - %	25 to 100 (*4 studies 100%*)	8
Work-related injuries - %	3 to 15	4
Sports/leisure-related injuries - %	14, 28	2
Terror-related injuries - %	50	1
Other/not defined	14 to 30	5
Presence of pain or mental health disorders other than PTSD (Studies not reporting n=17)		
Pain, including headaches - %	11 to 100 (*1 study 100%*)	5
Depression and/or depressive symptoms - %	9 to 90	8
Substance use disorders - %	14 to 42	3
Anxiety disorders other than PTSD or anxiety symptoms unspecified - %	9 to 60	3
Obsessive-compulsive disorder - %	15, 100 (*1 study 100%*)	2
Panic - %	14	1
Depression and anxiety disorders unspecified - %	71	1
Study type		
Cohort	28 to 307	14
Case-control	144	1
Cross-sectional	43 to 2525	15
Case series	10	1

* U.S. only

Prevalence of TBI/PTSD (Figures 2 and 3; Appendix D)

<u>*Reported prevalence of TBI/PTSD across study populations*</u>
Figure 2 displays the range of reported TBI/PTSD prevalence levels across study populations; studies involving U.S. military populations are listed first. As shown, the range of TBI/PTSD prevalence was broad (from 0% to 70%). Across all 31 published studies, plus the RAND study, the majority (n=22) reported prevalence levels of 20% or less. The few studies with values of 50% or more were small and/or had highly non-representative study populations (e.g., patients with obsessive-compulsive disorder).[53,65,73] Among the U.S. military/veteran studies, the three largest, most representative studies reported TBI/PTSD prevalence between 5% and 7%.[5,22,55] Each of these studies used similar self-report screening measures to assess both history of mTBI and current PTSD; thus, these numbers do not reflect actual diagnoses of mTBI or PTSD, which is almost certainly lower than the prevalence estimates based on the reported initial screening results. Among the four largest non-military studies, prevalence ranged from 8% to 30%.[58,59,63,67] Two of these studies involved populations that were comprised entirely of individuals with a history of TBI.[58,63] The other two involved clinic/hospital cohorts, identified diagnoses that were mostly mild and moderate TBI, and assessed for PTSD using a structured clinical interview (e.g., Clinician-administered PTSD Scale [CAPS], Structured Clinical Interview for the DSM-IV [SCID]) which are considered to be more stringent than the frequently used self-report PTSD screening measures (e.g., PTSD Checklist [PCL], Impact of Events Scale [IES]). Both of these studies reported TBI/PTSD prevalence of 8% in their study populations.[59,67]

Figure 2. Prevalence of TBI/PTSD across study populations

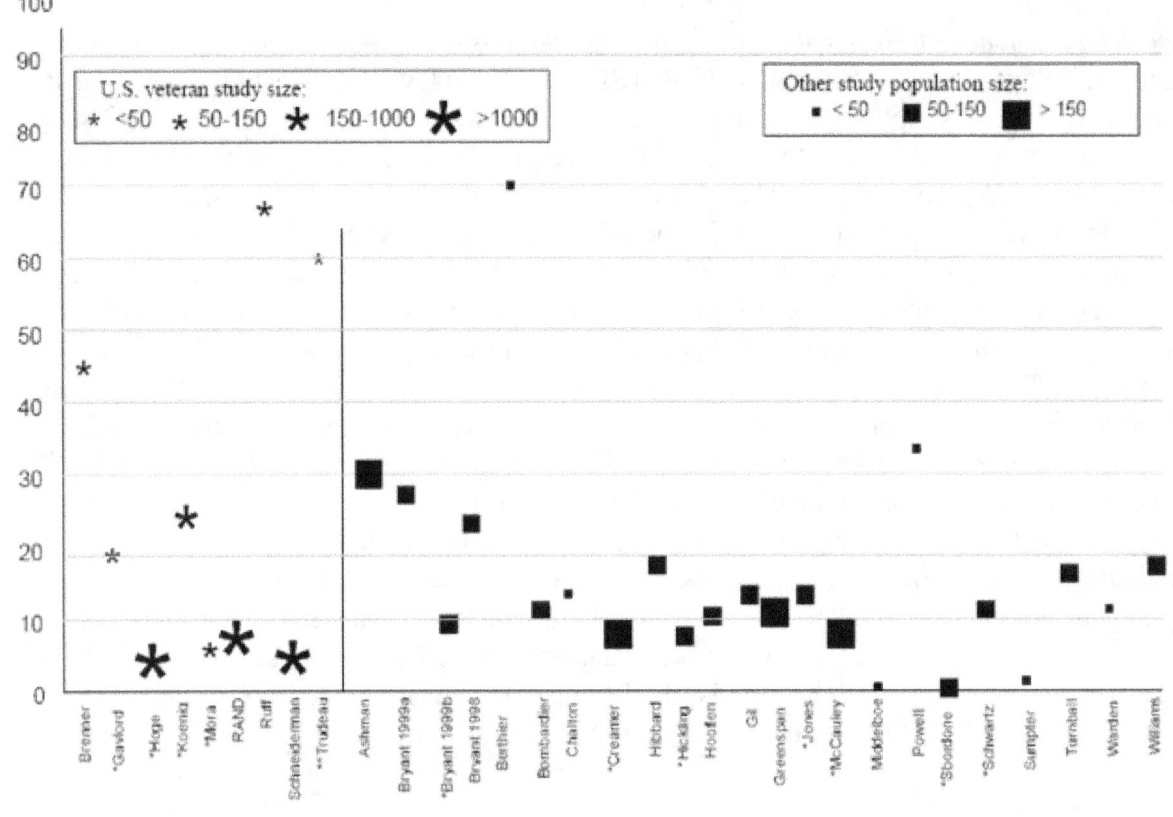

* Study populations included participants with and without TBI history. Unless indicated, all other study populations were comprised exclusively of participants with TBI history.
** Study population was comprised exclusively of participants with PTSD.

Reported prevalence of TBI/PTSD by level of TBI severity

Prevalence of TBI/PTSD may differ by TBI severity. In the studies that involved study populations that were homogenous by TBI severity, or that reported PTSD prevalence stratified by TBI severity, prevalence of PTSD ranged from 0% to 89% in participants with a history of mTBI,[21,22,52,53,55,57,59-61,65,67-70,75,76,79-81] 8% to 55% for those with a history of moderate TBI,[57,65,67,74,75,79,80] and 0% to 19% for those with a history of severe TBI.[57,61,64-66,79,80] Because the emphasis of this evidence review was on mTBI, we were particularly interested in prevalence of PTSD among individuals with a history of mTBI. Figure 3 depicts the prevalence of mTBI/PTSD across studies, again listing studies of U.S. military and veteran populations first. It is important to emphasize the different denominator used in the prevalence values reported in Figure 3 (# with mTBI/PTSD / # of individuals with mTBI) in contrast to Figure 2 (# with TBI/PTSD / # of individuals in study *with or without* TBI).

Two points should be noted when examining the studies in this way. First, when restricting the denominator to individuals with a positive history of mTBI, we are asking a slightly different question about prevalence. In Figure 2, we examine prevalence of TBI/PTSD across entire study populations while, in Figure 3, we examine prevalence of PTSD in individuals with a history of mTBI. Both questions were of interest for this review. However, when examining prevalence of PTSD among individuals with a history of mTBI, the reported prevalence values tend to be higher, which could be due to differential exposure among these individuals or other selection biases. Note that some values in Figure 3 are the same as in Figure 2 because these studies involved populations in which all participants had a history of mTBI.[21,22,52,53,55,59,60,61,68,69,70,76]

Second, the prevalence of PTSD in U.S. military/veteran study populations with a history of mTBI tends to look somewhat higher than prevalence of PTSD in the civilian study populations; however, the assessment methods varied and could account for these differences. The two large U.S. military studies reported PTSD prevalence levels of 33% and 39% among those with a history of mTBI.[22,55] These values are consistent with the findings of the RAND study, which reported a PTSD prevalence of 34% among those with history of TBI (note that the RAND study was not exclusive to mTBI though likely predominantly identified mTBI).[5] Each of these studies used similar self-report screening measures for both mTBI and PTSD; thus, these numbers do not reflect actual diagnoses of mTBI or PTSD. In contrast to these studies, the largest of the civilian studies reported PTSD prevalence between 12% and 27%.[59,60,67,68,70] While lower than prevalence values in the military/veteran studies, all five of these studies involved patients specifically treated for trauma in a hospital or clinic and utilized a structured clinical interview to assess PTSD. No studies provided estimates of mTBI/PTSD prevalence in civilians who were not specifically treated in a hospital or clinic for TBI.

Figure 3. Prevalence of PTSD among study participants with a history of mTBI

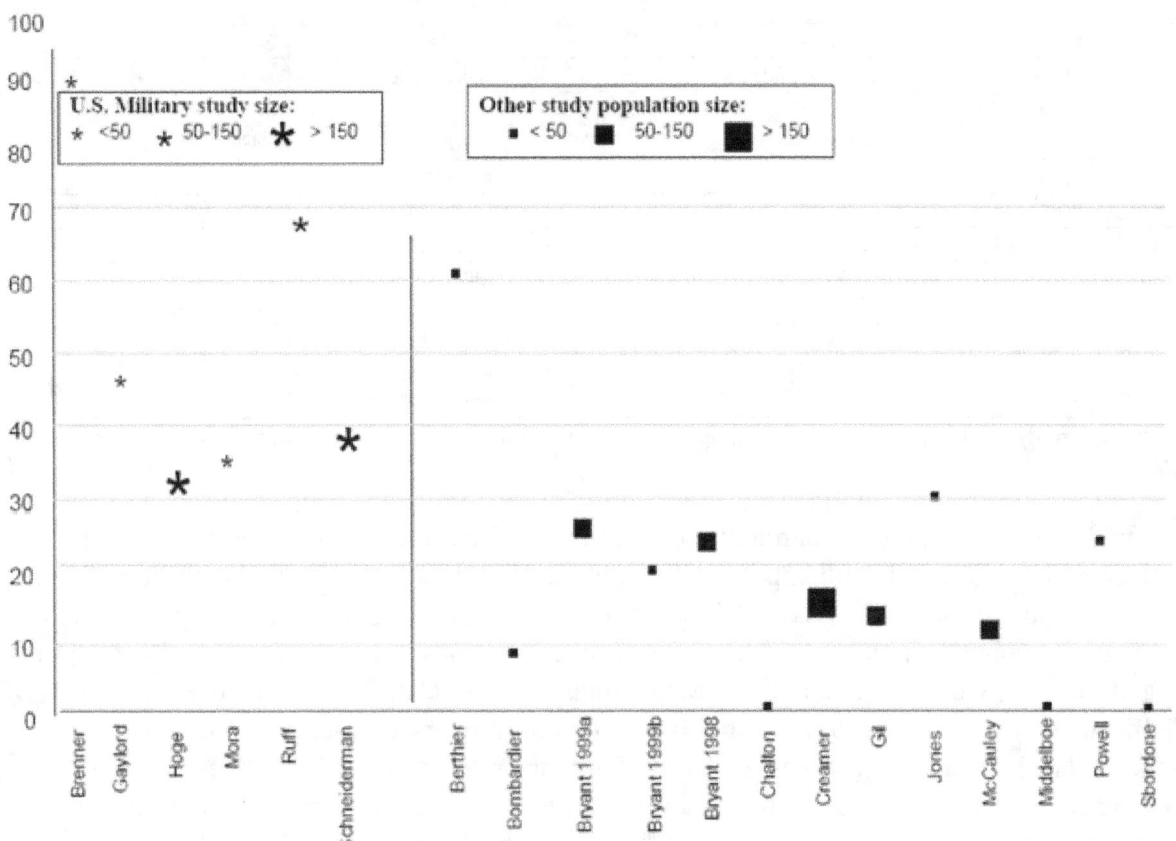

Reported prevalence of TBI/PTSD by trauma etiology
In addition to variation by TBI severity, prevalence of TBI/PTSD would be expected to vary by important exposure characteristics including type of trauma, time since trauma exposure, and number of trauma exposures. Most studies described populations with diverse trauma sources. To examine potential differences in TBI/PTSD prevalence by military versus non-military etiologies, we compared studies that reported prevalence of PTSD in populations with TBI, if they: 1) reported prevalence explicitly by etiology; or 2) reported prevalence in populations in which ≥75% had a single etiology. The following table lists these studies organized by military and non-military etiology. We use the term 'military' and further describe the percent by etiology of blast or burn (presumed combat) because in some instances military trauma may not be due to direct combat injuries (e.g., non-combat motor vehicle crashes). All the military-related studies identified in this table, except Koenigs et al.,[54] involved personnel serving in OEF/OIF.

Table 2. Prevalence of PTSD among individuals with TBI, by trauma etiology

Author, year	Injury etiology	TBI severity	% of TBI subjects with PTSD
Military-related Injuries			
Gaylord et al., 2008[52]	Military, blast and burn (100%)	Mild 100%	45%
Hoge et al., 2008[22]	Military, blast (75%)	Mild 100%	33%
Koenigs et al., 2008[54]	Military (100%)	Penetrating 100%	32%
Mora et al., 2009[81]	Military, blast and burn (100%)	Mild 95% Severe 5%	35%
RAND, 2008[5]	Military (100%)	Not Reported	34%
Ruff et al., 2008[53]	Military, blast (100%)	Mild 100%	66%
Non-military injuries*			
Bryant et al., 1998[70]	Motor Vehicle Crashes (MVC) (100%)	Mild 100%	24%
Bryant et al., 1999b[71]	MVC (100%)	Mild 100%	20%
Gil et al., 2005[60]	MVC (84%)	Mild 100%	14%
Hickling et al., 1998[72]	MVC (100%)	Not reported	56%
Jones et al., 2005[61]	MVC (100%)	Mild 100%	32% at time 1 19% at time 2
Schwartz et al. 2007[56]	MVC (82%)	Mild 32% Moderate 21% Severe 47%	42%

* Excluded 1 study reporting TBI/PTSD among a population of patients with obsessive-compusive disorder (Berthier et al., 2001)[65]

This table contains data points similar to those in Figure 3 except that all levels of TBI severity are included. Of note is that other potentially important parameters also varied considerably (e.g., study size and representativeness, PTSD assessment method, time since trauma exposure). Not taking into account the potential effects of these other variables, the prevalence of TBI/PTSD ranged from 32% to 66% in individuals with military-related TBI.[5,22,52-54,81] The prevalence of TBI/PTSD ranged from 14% to 56% in individuals with non-military injuries.[56,60,61,69,70,72] As opposed to the studies in which subjects had a history of military-related TBI, all of which reported PTSD prevalence greater than 30%, four of the seven reports involving subjects with non-military injuries reported values less than 30%.[60,61,69,70] Whether this is an epidemiologically important difference is not certain, as other study parameters may have simultaneously affected results.

Reported prevalence of TBI/PTSD by time since trauma

Similar to trauma type, time since trauma was widely variable across studies and even within studies. Across this group of studies, the potential effect of time since trauma on TBI/PTSD prevalence would best be described in three longitudinal studies enrolling patients with a TBI and assessing for PTSD at different time points post-injury. Unfortunately, no patterns could be discerned. Jones et al. identified PTSD in 32% of patients with TBI history at six weeks post-injury, and in 19% at three months post-injury.[61] Greenspan et al. identified PTSD in 11% of patients with TBI history at six months post-injury, and in 16% at twelve months post-injury.[58] Bryant and Harvey reported PTSD in 24% of patients with TBI history at six months post-injury, and 22% at two years post-injury.[70]

Reported prevalence of TBI/PTSD by methods of assessment

Studies varied in terms of how a positive screen or diagnosis for PTSD was defined and in how TBI was assessed and defined. Methods of PTSD assessment included structured interviews, self-report instruments, and non-standardized diagnoses by clinicians. Overall, within studies utilizing structured interviews (e.g., CAPS and SCID) to assess PTSD, prevalence of TBI/PTSD ranged from 3% to 70% across study populations.[54,59,60,62,63,65,67-72,74,78-80] For studies utilizing self-report instruments (e.g., PCL and IES), prevalence of TBI/PTSD ranged from 5% to 66%.[5,22,52,53,55,57,58,64,76,81] One study reported a 10% prevalence of diagnosed TBI/PTSD using the PTSD Inventory; however, it was unclear whether the instrument was used as a self-report instrument or as a structured interview.[66] Finally, one study did not articulate how PTSD was defined or diagnosed; this study reported no cases of PTSD among patients with a history of TBI.[21] Structured clinical interviews, particularly the CAPS, are considered the gold-standard for PTSD assessment and diagnosis. The studies that used the CAPS to assess PTSD identified prevalence levels of TBI/PTSD ranging from 3% to 38%.[59,60,62,72,78,80] Among the studies using the SCID, prevalence ranged from 8% to 44% across entire study populations.[54,63,65,67,71,79]

Self-report measures, including instruments used for screening, are considered less valid methods for PTSD assessment. Studies that utilized the PTSD Checklist (PCL) to assess for PTSD used different score thresholds to define the presence of PTSD. Studies did not present results in a fashion that would allow for calculation of prevalence at a single common value. The prevalence of TBI/PTSD ranged from 33% to 66% using a cut score of 50 (3 studies),[22,53,55] and 35% to 45% using a cut score of 44 (2 studies).[52,81] Each of the four studies using the Impact of Events Scale (IES) involved participants with a positive history of TBI. Using a cutoff of 35, Greenspan and colleagues reported a prevalence of 11% six months after injury and a prevalence of 16% twelve months after injury.[58] Two studies used a cutoff of 26 and reported prevalence levels of 18% and 34%.[64,75] Lastly, Middelboe and colleagues reported that no participants with TBI diagnoses "fulfilled the DSM-III-R criteria for post-traumatic stress disorder," but 11% had "moderate" or higher scores on the IES.[76]

Methods of identifying TBI cases also varied widely across studies. Frequently, survey study participants were asked questions varying by study to assess a positive history of TBI.[5,21,22,55,63,64,73] Alternatively, participants were recruited from hospitals following treatment for trauma or, specifically, head injury. These patients' TBI history was obtained from medical records alone or a combination of medical records review supplemented by questionnaire.[52,53,56-62,65-70,72,74-76,78,79-81] As a result, systematically examining prevalence of TBI/PTSD by method of TBI assessment was not possible.

Key Question #2.

#2a What is known about the relative accuracy of diagnostic tests used for assessing mild TBI when comorbid with PTSD?

#2b What is known about the relative accuracy of diagnostic tests used for assessing PTSD when comorbid with mild TBI?

Summary of Findings

There were no published studies addressing the relative accuracy of diagnostic tests used for assessing mTBI history or current PTSD when one condition co-occurs with the other.

Secondary Findings

One study compared the relative accuracy of four PTSD assessment tools in a cohort of individuals with a history of severe TBI. A sub-study involving the same population of individuals qualitatively explored reasons for false positive PTSD diagnoses when using a self-report assessment tool versus a structured clinical interview.

Details of Studies – Secondary Findings

Comparison of PTSD assessment tools in individuals with a history of severe TBI

One single-center small study compared four diagnostic measures of PTSD in individuals who had been diagnosed with severe TBI (defined as history of post-traumatic amnesia for more than one day).[62] Results varied widely depending on the measures used. Authors administered two self-report measures of PTSD, the IES and the Post-traumatic Diagnostic Scale (PDS), and a structured clinical interview measure for PTSD, the CAPS, to a convenience sample of 34 civilians whose severe TBI event had occurred at least three months prior to the study (Table 3). Four sets of criteria were used to define cases of PTSD: 1) IES scores > 25; 2) fulfillment of PDS criteria B-F; 3) fulfillment of CAPS criteria B-F; and 4) fulfillment of CAPS criteria B-F *plus* a clinician's judgment that the endorsed symptoms were valid and indeed related to trauma. The latter two criteria were referred to as "CAPS-without clinical judgment" and "CAPS-with clinical judgment," respectively. Participants were primarily male (88%), were aged 20-60 years (mean=34; SD=11), and had 10-20 years of formal education (mean=12; SD=2). The sources of injury were motor vehicle crashes (47%), falls (32%), assaults (18%), and sports activities (3%).

Fulfillment of CAPS-with clinical judgment was considered the gold-standard PTSD diagnostic tool in this study. Only one individual (3%) met criteria for PTSD based on this assessment tool. Six individuals (18%) met criteria based on CAPS-without clinical judgment, 15 (44%) met criteria based on the IES, and 20 (59%) met criteria based on the PDS. Both self-report questionnaires (IES and PDS) identified significantly more (p<0.05) false positive PTSD cases than CAPS-without clinical judgment. There were no false negative cases identified by the IES or PDS; all cases identified by CAPS-without clinical judgment were also identified by these self-report questionnaires. Therefore, based on the definitions used by these authors, this study supports the use of the IES and PDS self-report questionnaires as screening tools for PTSD among individuals with severe TBI. However, structured clinical interviews were deemed the most appropriate diagnostic tool for diagnosis of PTSD after severe TBI. There was indication that individuals may have mistaken their TBI-related symptoms for PTSD symptoms on the self-report questionnaires, with these discrepancies becoming clear only during the process of structured clinical interview. Clinical judgment thus provided the opportunity for differential diagnosis of PTSD versus symptoms of severe TBI based on the context of the symptoms as well as potentially confounding factors.

Potential reasons for false positive PTSD diagnoses in individuals with a history of severe TBI
One qualitative study was conducted by the same authors as above and explored reasons for false positive PTSD diagnoses when using a self-report assessment tool (PDS) as compared to a structured clinical interview (CAPS) as the "gold-standard" assessment method.[35] The study population consisted of the same 34 civilians with a severe TBI history; however, the sole individual diagnosed with PTSD using the CAPS-with clinical judgment was excluded so as to examine PTSD symptoms that were reported by individuals without PTSD.

Self-reported and clinician-rated PTSD symptoms (PDS versus CAPS) were compared by DSM-IV PTSD symptoms clusters: re-experiencing, avoidance, and hyperarousal. Based on the PDS, 91% of participants reported two or more hyperarousal symptoms, 78% reported three or more avoidance symptoms, and 67% reported at least one re-experiencing symptom. Only one PTSD symptom (insomnia) was reported in more than 20% of participants when using the CAPS. Using a standardized interview prompt to explore the identified discrepancies, investigators found that cognitive impairments, misunderstanding of self-report items, and true symptoms overlap seemed to lead to endorsement of PTSD symptoms on the PDS. For example, individuals with loss of memory for their traumatic event confused "curiosity" about their event for "re-experiencing" the event. While symptoms may have been reported as "intrusive," they were not found to be accompanied by fear or emotional distress. Additionally, while participants frequently endorsed "having upsetting thoughts," these thoughts were often associated with the effects of the severe TBI and not with the trauma itself. Similarly, avoidance-related questions (e.g., loss of interest, detachment, or reduction in affect) were frequently endorsed in relation to functional difficulties associated with the severe TBI rather than the traumatic event. Endorsement of hyperarousal symptoms often had to do with individuals having to cope with cognitive and physical impairments and fear of re-injury. In all, this study highlights the overlap and potential confusion around assessment of symptoms of PTSD and symptoms related to a TBI.

Table 3. Secondary findings for Key Question 2: Assessment of PTSD in individuals with severe TBI

Study / Country	Study design and population	n	Characteristics of participants	Traumatic brain injury definition/measure	Post-traumatic stress disorder assessment	% of subjects fulfilling criteria for PTSD
Sumpter 2005;[62] Sumpter 2006[35] United Kingdom	Cross-sectional Subjects recruited from community outpatient and rehabilitation services, and volunteer organizations	n=34; all TBI	*Data for all study subjects* Trauma etiology: MVC 47%; fall 32%; assault 18%; sports injury 3% TBI severity: severe 100% Time of assessment or since trauma: 6 years (0.6-34) Mean age (range): 40 (20-60) Women: 12% Race: NR Education: NR Pain: NR Mental health disorders other than PTSD: NR	Not reported, subjects with severe TBI history recruited from community outpatient and rehabilitation services and voluntary organizations.	Compared 4 assessment tools: 1) Post-traumatic Diagnostic Scale (PDS), based on DSM-IV criteria, criteria B-F fulfilled 2) Impact of Event Scale questionnaire (IES), total score > 25 = "case" 3) Clinician-Administered PTSD Scale (CAPS), without clinical judgment, criteria B-F fulfilled 4) CAPS, with clinical judgment, criteria B-F fulfilled	1) PDS: 59% (n=20) 2) IES: 44% (n=15) 3) CAPS w/o clinical judgment: 18% (n=6) 4) CAPS with clinical judgment: 3% (n=1)

Key Question #3.

#3a Are there psychosocial or pharmacological therapies used for treatment of mTBI and PTSD simultaneously?

#3b Are therapies for treatment of mTBI effective when mTBI is comorbid with PTSD? Is there evidence of harms?

#3c Are therapies for treatment of PTSD effective when PTSD is comorbid with mTBI? Is there evidence of harms?

Summary of Findings:

3A: We found no randomized or non-randomized controlled clinical trials, systematic reviews, cohort studies, case control studies, or cross-sectional studies that discussed psychosocial or pharmacological therapies designed to simultaneously treat symtpoms of mTBI and PTSD.

3B: We found no randomized or non-randomized controlled clinical trials, systematic reviews, cohort studies, case control studies, or cross-sectional studies that examined the effectivess of treatments for mTBI symptoms when patients had PTSD.

3C: We found no randomized or non-randomized controlled clinical trials, systematic reviews, cohort studies, case control studies, or cross-sectional studies that examined the effectivess of treatments for PTSD when patients had a history of mTBI.

Secondary Findings:

One small, single-center, good-quality randomized controlled trial examined the efficacy of a cognitive-behavioral treatment for individuals with acute stress disorder (ASD) and a history of mTBI. The study found that patients who received cognitive-behavioral therapy developed PTSD at a lower rate than those who received supportive therapy.

Two case reports discussed treatment approaches that utilized empirically supported therapies to treat individuals with mTBI history and current PTSD.

Details of Studies – Secondary Findings

Treatment of mTBI and Acute Stress Disorder

One small, good quality study examined the comparative efficacy of cognitive-behavior therapy (CBT) and supportive therapy in reducing symptoms and preventing the development of PTSD in 24 civilians with history of mTBI and current acute stress disorder (ASD; Table 4).[82] ASD is a post-traumatic stress reaction that occurs within the first month post-trauma. The symptoms are similar to PTSD, with the exception that individuals with ASD must also experience symptoms of dissociation. Previous research has shown that approximately 80% of people with ASD go on to develop PTSD.[83]

This randomized controlled trial enrolled men and women who had experienced either a motor vehicle crash or nonsexual assault within the preceding two weeks. In order to be eligible, patients must have met criteria for ASD, as determined by the Acute Stress Disorder Interview, and mTBI, which was defined as post-traumatic amnesia of less than 24 hours and a Glasgow Coma Scale score of 13-15. Those randomized to CBT received five weekly 90-minute sessions that included psychoeducation, progressive muscle relaxation, imaginal exposure to the traumatic event, cognitive restructuring, and in vivo exposure to avoided stimuli. Patients in the supportive counseling condition also received five weekly 90-minute sessions, comprised of psychoeducation and problem-solving skills. There was no mention of modificiations made to the therapy protocols due to potential cognitive impairments in the study participants.

Immediately post-treatment, PTSD was less prevalent in the CBT group (8%; n=1) than the supportive therapy group (58%; n=7). At the six-month follow-up, 17% (n=2) of the CBT group and 58% (n=7) of the supportive therapy group met criteria for PTSD. Further, at post-treatment and six-month follow-up, patients in the CBT condition experienced large, significant decreases in PTSD symptomology (as measured by both the IES and CAPS). Both groups experienced a moderate decrease in depressive symptoms at post-treatment and a small decrease at six-month follow-up, but there was not a statistically significant difference between the groups. The authors concluded that CBT is effective in reducing symptoms and preventing onset of PTSD in patients with ASD and mTBI history.

Case studies reporting on the treatment of patients with mTBI/PTSD
Two case reports (one involving a U.S. military patient) presented information regarding the treatment of mTBI symptoms and PTSD in individual patients (Table 4).[84,85] In both case reports, the therapist used cognitive-behavioral techniques to treat the symptoms of PTSD (cognitive processing therapy; exposure and cognitive restructuring) with few modifications. To manage mTBI-related symptoms, the therapists encouraged the patients to use compensatory strategies (e.g., using personal digital assistants, scheduling cognitive breaks). Both reports highlighted the range of problems experienced by the individuals they were treating (e.g., anger, depression, substance abuse) and advocated for an idiographic, integrative approach. These case studies reported a decrease in symptoms of anxiety and depression; however, significant residual symptoms remained.

Table 4. Secondary findings for Key Question 3: Treatment of mTBI/PTSD

Study / Country / Study design	# Subjects; % Dropout / Lost to follow-up	Subjects	Method of assessment	Treatment	Duration of therapy	Treatment outcomes	Study quality
Bryant 2003[82] Australia Randomized Controlled Trial (RCT)	n=24	Mean age (range): 31 (18 - 60) Women: 67% Race: NR Trauma etiology: motor vehicle crash (MVC) or non-sexual assault Pain: NR Other mental health conditions: NR	TBI: Glasgow Coma Scale PTSD: Impact of Event Scale (IES) and Clinician Administered PTSD Scale (CAPS)	1. Cognitive Behavior Therapy (CBT) Group (n=12) 2. Supportive Counseling (SC) Group (n=12)	6 mos	<u>Mean CAPS scores (SD)</u> Baseline CBT: 65.42 (10.60) SC: 62.42 (14.58) Frequency subscale a. Post-treatment CBT: 13.50 (10.24) SC: 23.83 (15.30); p=0.002 b. 6 mos follow-up CBT: 16.83 (13.04) SC: 25.25 (16.21); p=0.03 Intensity subscale a. Post-treatment CBT: 12.00 (9.71) SC: 21.33 (12.49); p=0.003 b. 6 mos follow-up CBT: 14.62 (9.12) SC: 24.50 (13.13); p=0.02 <u>Subjects meeting PTSD criteria:</u> a. Post-treatment CBT: 8% (n=1) SC: 58% (n=7); p<0.05 b. 6 mos follow-up CBT: 17% (n=2) SC: 58% (n=7); p<0.05	Good

Batten 2008[84] U.S. Case Report	1	24 year old, Caucasian male Trauma etiology: Combat Pain: joint pain and headaches Other mental health conditions: depression, alcohol abuse, marijuana abuse	TBI: Clinic diagnosis, criteria unknown PTSD: Clinician Administered PTSD Scale (CAPS) & PTSD Checklist (PCL)	Cognitive processing therapy; two sessions outlining behavioral activation for depression & sleep hygiene; one session on decreasing substance abuse; addressed memory compensation strategies with polytrauma team	19 individual therapy sessions	Lost PTSD diagnosis, although still had significant symptoms; decreased symptoms of depression; decreased alcohol use; marijuana abstinence	Poor
McGrath 1997[85] England Case Report	1	33 year old male Race: NR Trauma etiology: MVC Pain: Ear pain and headaches Other mental health conditions: NR	TBI: Head injury with PTA of 40 minutes PTSD: Clinical interview used to determine DSM-IV criteria	Progressive muscle relaxation; anger management; cognitive restructuring; graded in vivo exposure; response prevention for checking behaviors; compensatory cognitive strategies; supportive therapy	NR	Slight decrease in anxiety symptoms; decrease in anger; decrease in symptoms of depression; no change in subjective cognitive symptoms, but improved work functioning	Poor

LITERATURE REVIEW KQ 1-3 - LIMITATIONS

The existing literature has several limitations. The quality of identified studies was generally fair and external validity was generally poor. Few prevalence studies were actually population-based. Most were small and conducted in a single medical or research center. Authors frequently only recruited individuals who had been hospitalized or received medical attention specifically for their trauma. No large studies representative of the entire OEF/OIF veteran population have been conducted using currently implemented screening and diagnostic tools. Therefore, the applicability of the current literature to existing populations of interest, screened and diagnosed with currently utilized tools, is not known. By extension, the true prevalence of TBI/PTSD, particularly mTBI/PTSD, is not known. Reported findings from most studies likely overestimate the prevalence of TBI/PTSD, especially mTBI/PTSD, in the populations of interest. For example, civilian individuals recruited from emergency departments likely represent more severe, more symptomatic cases of TBI (and PTSD) than individuals who experience a TBI for which they do not seek medical attention. Assessment instruments, ascertainment methods, timing, and diagnostic criteria used to identify TBI and PTSD cases varied widely. Different methods and thresholds to define disease and injury can have profound impact on the prevalence, severity, natural history and response to treatment of a condition. This may be particularly relevant where individual responses may be affected by the potential for compensation. Study populations were heterogeneous and results were rarely reported according to key clinical characteristics of interest (e.g., age, gender, race, socioeconomic status, trauma etiology or time, presence of pain or mental health disorders other than PTSD) that may have an impact on prevalence estimates. We attempted to minimize publication bias by using broad search terms and multiple databases, and by seeking input from our Technical Advisory Panel members and external peer reviewers (including consensus panel members). We included the large RAND study,[5] even though it may not technically meet definitions for peer-reviewed publications.

ACTIVE RESEARCH

Summary of Findings

Although there are a number of ongoing, active research studies that include patients with TBI/PTSD, few will specifically address the key questions identified for this report.

Details of Findings

The ongoing studies, sorted by key question, are summarized in Appendix E, Tables 1-3. We identified seven studies that will provide information about the prevalence of TBI/PTSD (Table 1). Six of the studies include OEF and/or OIF soldiers or veterans. Sample sizes vary widely; the largest study intends to assess TBI history and PTSD in up to 60,000 veterans. The methods of assessment of TBI history and PTSD vary and include chart review, self report, symptom checklists, and structured diagnostic interviews.

We identified eight studies that will provide information related to the assessment of mTBI/PTSD (Table 2). Three of the studies will also address key question #1 and are included in Appendix E, Table 1. All but one of the studies include military personnel, with reported sample sizes ranging from 120 to 850. The methods of assessment are largely similar to those reported in Table 1, although magnetic resonance imaging, sleep studies, neuroendocrine measures, and a smell test are also being used.

Six studies were identified that examine treatments for symptoms of mTBI/PTSD. Five of the studies include OEF/OIF veterans or their family members; the remaining study will likely include veterans. Reported sample sizes range from 6 to 300. Treatments to be evaluated include psychotherapy, psychiatric and sleep medications, relaxation therapy, sleep education, support teams, and hyperbaric oxygen therapy. One of the studies is a randomized, controlled trial.

ACTIVE RESEARCH - LIMITATIONS

Our reporting of active research is based solely on responses obtained from individuals who received our request for information and chose to respond. No follow-up contact was made with non-responders. Thus, there may be other ongoing studies pertinent to our key questions that were not identified by this process. Most ongoing studies we identified are not enrolling broad-based populations of individuals to estimate population prevalence of TBI/PTSD (especially mTBI/PTSD). We did not identify any studies that attempt to compare the diagnostic accuracy of different assessment tools for identification of TBI history or current PTSD when the conditions co-occur (especially for individuals likely to have mTBI/PTSD). We identified only one ongoing randomized and controlled treatment trial. Future research needs to incorporate these items to ensure that the key questions covered in this review can be addressed.

The studies listed in Appendix E all include at least some patients with TBI/PTSD. Given the ongoing nature of the studies, it was not always possible to identify the exact proportion of patients who would have TBI/PTSD or the severity of the TBI experienced by the patients.

SUMMARY AND DISCUSSION

Our findings indicate that reported prevalence of TBI/PTSD varies widely. Differences in populations, study methodology, trauma severity and etiology, and methods and definitions of ascertainment weaken the strength of the evidence and do not permit accurate prevalence estimates, particularly for patient subgroups of greatest interest to the Department of Veterans Affairs. The three largest studies involving U.S. military personnel and veterans of OEF/OIF, while based on different study populations and survey methods, had relatively consistent results. Results of these three studies indicated that TBI/PTSD (the majority in the RAND study likely to have mTBI/PTSD) occurred in approximately 5% to 7% of individuals. Among individuals who reported a history of probable TBI, probable PTSD was identified in 33% to 39%. Prevalence varied widely in other studies, likely due to different methods to define and identify cases of TBI and PTSD. We emphasize that these factors can have a profound impact on estimates for prevalence, severity, natural history, and response to treatment for these conditions. In particular, methods that utilize highly sensitive but less specific screening instruments that incorporate self-reported outcomes that can be influenced by financial compensation are likely to increase prevalence estimates and over-diagnose individuals with milder conditions. These points are evidenced by the recent commentary and letters of response published in the *New England Journal of Medicine*.[23,28] Similarly, studies that enroll subjects hospitalized or receiving medical care specifically for their trauma are likely to overestimate prevalence. Because these individuals may differ substantially in many ways (both known and unknown) from individuals with less severe TBI/PTSD and/or cases detected through other screening methods/thresholds, caution should be taken when extrapolating findings from one population to another.

We were unable to identify any studies that evaluated the accuracy of diagnostic tests for individuals with suspected mTBI/PTSD. Furthermore, we were unable to identify any randomized controlled trials and only two case reports related to efficacy of treatment specifically for mTBI/PTSD. Therefore, there is insufficient evidence required to make high quality diagnostic and treatment recommendations pertinent to our key questions. While we identified a large number of ongoing studies related to TBI and PTSD, none are likely to provide high-quality, direct evidence pertaining to key questions 2 and 3 (methods of assessment and treatment). We have provided some recommendations below for the general design, conduct, and outcome measurements for future research studies.

CONCLUSIONS

The reported prevalence of TBI/PTSD varies widely, likely depending on patient characteristics, trauma etiology, disease definition, and ascertainment method. There is no information on the diagnostic accuracy of commonly used tests to assess history of mTBI or current PTSD when both conditions are present. There is no information on the effectiveness and harms of therapies in adults with mTBI/PTSD. There is considerable on-going research in this area. However, long-term prospective observational studies are needed that use standardized, validated measures of TBI (particularly mTBI) history and PTSD to determine TBI/PTSD prevalence, severity, and outcomes. Among military personnel, pre-deployment as well as post-deployment assessment should be obtained using objective measures that limit ascertainment, recall, or reporting bias. Outcomes according to clinically-relevant patient characteristics, trauma etiology and subtypes, and time from trauma are required. Diagnostic accuracy studies are needed that utilize established quality methods as reported in the STARD initiative[47] and recommended in the QUADAS report.[86] Adequately powered, high-quality randomized, controlled treatment trials in populations of interest are required to evaluate the clinical effectiveness and harms of potential therapeutic options, especially among individuals with mTBI/PTSD.

FUTURE RESEARCH RECOMMENDATIONS

Long-term prospective observational studies are needed that use standardized and validated measures of TBI history and PTSD to determine prevalence, severity, and outcomes of TBI/PTSD. There is a clear need for researchers to come to consensus on the definitions and measures that will be used consistently across studies in order to facilitate comparison of results. Among military personnel, pre-deployment as well as post-deployment assessment should be obtained using objective measures that limit ascertainment, recall, or reporting bias. Outcomes according to clinically relevant patient characteristics, trauma etiology and severity, and time from trauma are required. Diagnostic accuracy studies are needed that utilize established quality methods such as QUADAS. Randomized controlled treatment trials in populations of interest are required to evaluate the effectiveness and harms of potential therapeutic options, especially among individuals with mTBI/PTSD. Research specific to care coordination and treatment planning between specialty clinics and providers should also be considered.

Future research should be devoted to addressing these question using more representative samples and longitudinal methods. Methodologically, we recommend that future research in this area adhere to guidelines for reporting observational studies as report in the Strengthening the Reporting of Observational Studies in Epidemiology (STROBE) Statement.[87] As most research relies on samples with probable TBI history recruited from hospital settings, future investigations should include both nationally representative samples, as well as specific samples of interest, such as OEF/OIF veterans or populations seeking services primarily for trauma exposure (e.g., those seeking mental health services, victims' advocacy, or legal services as victims of crime). Future research should develop innovative methods to obtain information necessary for assessing the occurrence of TBI near the time of injury without relying on subject recall or hospital admission to identify patient populations, especially given the suspected low rates at which those with potential mTBI seek emergency medical treatment.

Research optimizing the diagnostic accuracy of assessment for both TBI history and current PTSD in representative populations using gold-standard assessments is of paramount importance. Accuracy is contingent upon research clarifying diagnostic debates regarding how to best assess these conditions when they co-occur. Additionally, little is known regarding the trajectory of symptoms over time for those with either TBI history or current PTSD, and whether outcomes differ among individuals classified as having mTBI/PTSD versus those with just PTSD (especially after controlling for potentially confounding variables). Longitudinal research is needed to assess the degree of overlap in these conditions and long-term outcomes using gold-standard instruments with increasing time from the traumatic event. Future research (and clinical care) would benefit from studies that adhere to the Standards for Reporting of Diagnostic Accuracy (STARD) statement.[47]

Finally, further research is needed that directly compares prevalence of TBI/PTSD among samples matched on important domains such as the type of traumatic events to which individuals were exposed (e.g., combat vs. MVC, physical assault, intimate partner violence), the number and severity of TBI events, demographic characteristics (e.g., gender, race, age), and methods of assessment. Results should be stratified by these clinical characteristics of interest. Furthermore, among military personnel, assessing symptomology prior to deployment and then immediately post-deployment could provide useful information regarding causation.

In regard to the treatment of PTSD among individuals with a history of mTBI, we recommend first evaluating the effectiveness of empirically supported treatments (ESTs) for PTSD (e.g., prolonged exposure therapy and cognitive processing therapy) among individuals with a history of mTBI. Ideally, individuals would be stratified by mTBI status (mTBI/PTSD vs. PTSD without mTBI), then randomized to either the EST or a minimal contact control condition. This design would enable researchers to examine the efficacy of the treatment among adults with mTBI/PTSD and to evaluate differential outcomes between participants with mTBI/PTSD and participants with PTSD but no mTBI history. If the two groups have equivalent outcomes on a variety of measures (PTSD symptomology, functioning, and quality of life), we recommend future research focus on improving outcomes for all individuals with PTSD, rather than focusing specifically on treatments for those with a history of mTBI. Within such a trial, we also suggest extracting treatment process data that would allow researchers to examine whether adults with mTBI/PTSD have more difficulty with tasks related to memory and attention (e.g., homework completion, engagement in imaginal exposure) than individuals with PTSD but no mTBI history. In the case of differential outcomes, such process data would allow researchers to begin to examine factors that may have contributed to lower levels of recovery among individuals with mTBI/PTSD. If memory or attentional problems do contribute to differential outcomes, we suggest the development and evaluation of a set of compensatory strategies that can be used in conjunction with existing ESTs to improve outcomes (e.g., the use of a personal digital assistant to remind individuals to complete homework and track anxiety levels). Of note, given the concentration difficulties associated with PTSD, such strategies may be benefecial for all veterans undergoing an EST for PTSD. Finally, if adding compensatory strategies to existing ESTs for PTSD does not improve outcomes among individuals with mTBI/PTSD, researchers should look to more substantially alter existing ESTs or begin to develop novel interventions.

REFERENCE LIST

1.　　Centers for Disease Control and Prevention. Traumatic brain injury in the United States: A report to Congress. Atlanta, GA: Centers for Disease Control and Prevention, 1999.

2.　　Institute of Medicine (IOM). Gulf war and health, Volume 7: Long-term consequences of traumatic brain injury. Washington, DC: The National Academies Press, 2009.

3.　　Warden D. Military TBI during the Iraq and Afghanistan wars. J Head Trauma Rehab 2006; 21(5):398-402.

4.　　Okie S. Traumatic brain injury in the war zone. N Engl J Med 2005; 352(20):2043-2047.

5.　　Tanielian T, Jaycox LH, Editors. Invisible wounds of war: Psychological and cognitive injuries, their consequences, and services to assist recovery. Santa Monica, CA: Rand Corporation, 2008. Available at: http://www.rand.org/pubs/monographs/MG720/.

6.　　Management of Concussion/mTBI Working Group. VA/DoD clinical practice guideline for management of concussion/mild traumatic brain injury. Washington DC: Department of Veterans Affairs and Department of Defense, 2009.

7.　　Gordon WA, Zafonte R, Cicerone K, Cantor J, Brown M, Lombard L, et al. Traumatic brain injury rehabilitation: state of the science. Am J Phys Med Rehab/Association of Academic Physiatrists 2006; 85(4):343-382.

8.　　American Psychiatric Association. Diagnostic and statistical manual of mental disorders. 4th ed., text revision ed. Washington, DC: American Psychiatric Association, 2000.

9.　　Kessler RC, Sonnega A, Bromet E, Hughes M, Nelson CB. Posttraumatic stress disorder in the National Comorbidity Survey. Arch Gen Psychiatry 1995; 52(12):1048-1060.

10.　　Resnick HS, Kilpatrick DG, Dansky BS, Saunders BE, Best CL. Prevalence of civilian trauma and posttraumatic stress disorder in a representative national sample of women. J Consult Clin Psychol 1993; 61(6):984-991.

11.　　Dohrenwend BP, Turner JB, Turse NA, Adams BG, Koenen KC, Marshall R. The psychological risks of Vietnam for U.S. veterans: A revisit with new data and methods. Science 2006; 313(5789):979-982.

12.　　Hoge CW, Terhakopian A, Castro CA, Messer SC, Engel CC. Association of posttraumatic stress disorder with somatic symptoms, health care visits, and absenteeism among Iraq war veterans. Am J Psychiatry 2007; 164(1):150-153.

13.　　Milliken CS, Auchterlonie JL, Hoge CW. Longitudinal assessment of mental health problems among active and reserve component soldiers returning from the Iraq war. JAMA-J Am Med Assoc 2007; 298(18):2141-2148.

14.　　Boscarino JA. Diseases among men 20 years after exposure to severe stress: Implications for clinical research and medical care. Psychosom Med 1997; 59(6):605-614.

15.   Boscarino JA, Chang J. Electrocardiogram abnormalities among men with stress-related psychiatric disorders: Implications for coronary heart disease and clinical research. Ann Behav Med 1999; 21(3):227-234.

16.   Kessler RC. Posttraumatic stress disorder: The burden to the individual and to society. J Clin Psychiatry 2000; 61(S5):4-12.

17.   Savoca E, Rosenheck R. The civilian labor market experiences of Vietnam-era veterans: The influence of psychiatric disorders. J Ment Health Policy Econ 2000; 3(4):199-207.

18.   Schnurr PP, Hayes AF, Lunney CA, McFall M, Uddo M. Longitudinal analysis of the relationship between symptoms and quality of life in veterans treated for posttraumatic stress disorder. J Consult Clin Psychol 2006; 74(4):707-713.

19.   Polusny, MA. Final Report for VA HSR&D Project RRP 08-252: Mild TBI/PTSD comorbidity and post-deployment outcomes in National Guard Soldiers. 2009. Abstract available at: http://www.hsrd.research.va.gov/research/abstracts.cfm?Project_ID=2141698843.

20.   Bryant RA, Hopwood S. Commentary on "Trauma to the Psyche and Soma." Cogn Behav Pract 2006; 13(1):17-23.

21.   Sbordone RJ, Liter JC. Mild traumatic brain injury does not produce post-traumatic stress disorder. Brain Inj 1995; 9(4):405-412.

22.   Hoge CW, McGurk D, Thomas JL, Cox AL, Engel CC, Castro CA. Mild traumatic brain injury in U.S. Soldiers returning from Iraq. N Engl J Med 2008; 358(5):453-463.

23.   Hoge CW, Goldberg HM, Castro CA. Care of war veterans with mild traumatic brain injury--flawed perspectives. N Engl J Med 2009; 360(16):1588-1591.

24.   Institute of Medicine. Gulf war and health: Volume 7. Long-term consequences of traumatic brain injury. December 4, 2008. Available at http://www.iom.edu/CMS/4683/60519.aspx.

25.   Kennedy JE, Jaffee MS, Leskin GA, Stokes JW, Leal FO, Fitzpatrick PJ. Posttraumatic stress disorder and posttraumatic stress disorder-like symptoms and mild traumatic brain injury. J Rehabil Res Dev 2007; 44(7):895-920.

26.   King NS. PTSD and traumatic brain injury: Folklore and fact? Brain Inj 2008; 22(1):1-5.

27.   Rogers JM, Read CA. Psychiatric comorbidity following traumatic brain injury. Brain Inj 2007; 21(13-14):1321-1333.

28.   Correspondence. Care of war veterans with mild traumatic brain injury. N Engl J Med 2009; 361(15):536-538.

29.   McMillan TM. Errors in diagnosing post-traumatic stress disorder after traumatic brain injury. Brain Inj 2001; 15(1):39-46.

30.   Kim E, Lauterbach EC, Reeve A, Arciniegas DB, Coburn KL, Mendez MF, et al. Neu-ropsychiatric complications of traumatic brain injury: a critical review of the literature (A report by the ANPA Committee on Research). J Neuropsych Clin Neurosci 2007; 19(2):106-127.

31.   Moore EL, Terryberry-Spohr L, Hope DA. Mild traumatic brain injury and anxiety seque-lae: A review of the literature. Brain Inj 2006; 20(2):117-132.

32.   O'Donnell ML, Creamer M, Bryant RA, Schnyder U, Shalev A. Posttraumatic disor-ders following injury: An empirical and methodological review. Clin Psychol Rev 2003; 23(4):587-603.

33.   Hiott DW, Labbate L. Anxiety disorders associated with traumatic brain injuries. Neu-roRehabilitation 2002; 17(4):345-355.

34.   Ohry A, Rattok J, Solomon Z. Post-traumatic stress disorder in brain injury patients. Brain Inj 1996; 10(9):687-695.

35.   Sumpter RE, McMillan TM. Errors in self-report of post-traumatic stress disorder after severe traumatic brain injury. Brain Inj 2006; 20(1):93-99.

36.   Cahill SP, Rothbaum BO, Resick PS, Follette VM. Cognitive-behavioral therapy for adults. In: Foa EB, Keane T.M., Friedman MJ, Cohen J.A., editors. Effective Treatments for PTSD: Practice Guidelines for the International Society for Traumatic Stress Studies. New York: Guilford Press, 2009: 139-222.

37.   Monson CM, Schnurr PP, Resick PS, Friedman MJ, Young-Xu Y, Stevens SP. Cognitive processing therapy for veterans with military-related posttraumatic stress disorder. J Con-sult Clin Psychol 2006; 74(5):898-907.

38.   Schnurr PP, Friedman MJ, Engel CC, Foa EB, Shea MT, Chow BK, et al. Cognitive behavioral therapy for posttraumatic stress disorder in women: A randomized controlled trial. JAMA-J Am Med Assoc 2007; 297(8):820-830.

39.   Rauch SA, Defever E, Favorite T, Duroe A, Garrity C, Martis B, et al. Prolonged expo-sure for PTSD in a Veterans Health Administration PTSD clinic. J Trauma Stress 2009; 22(1):60-64.

40.   Paniak C, Toller-Lobe G, Durand A, Nagy J. A randomized trial of two treatments for mild traumatic brain injury. Brain Inj 1998; 12(12):1011-1023.

41.   Paniak C, Toller-Lobe G, Reynolds S, Melnyk A, Nagy J. A randomized trial of two treat-ments for mild traumatic brain injury: 1 year follow-up. Brain Inj 2000; 14(3):219-226.

42.   Nampiaparampil DE. Prevalence of chronic pain after traumatic brain injury: A system-atic review. JAMA-J Am Med Assoc 2008; 300(6): 711-719.

43.   Carroll LJ, Cassidy JD, Holm L, Kraus J, Coronado VG. Methodological issues and re-search recommendations for mild traumatic brain injury: The WHO Collaborating Centre Task Force on Mild Traumatic Brain Injury. J Rehabil Med 2004; 43S:113-125.

44.　　American Psychiatric Association. Diagnostic and statistical manual of mental disorders. 3rd ed. Washington, DC: American Psychiatric Association, 1980.

45.　　American Psychiatric Association. Diagnostic and statistical manual of mental disorders. 3rd ed., revised ed. Washington, DC: American Psychiatric Association, 1987.

46.　　American Psychiatric Association. Diagnostic and statistical manual of mental disorders. 4th ed. Washington, DC: American Psychiatric Association, 1994.

47.　　Bossuyt PM, Reitsma JB, Bruns DE, Gatsonis CA, Glasziou PP, Irwig LM, et al. The STARD statement for reporting studies of diagnostic accuracy: Explanation and elaboration. Ann Intern Med 2003; 138(1):W1-12.

48.　　Leeflang MM, Deeks JJ, Gatsonis C, Bossuyt PM. Systematic reviews of diagnostic test accuracy. Ann Intern Med 2008; 149(12):889-897.

49.　　Harris RP, Helfand M, Woolf SH, Lohr KN, Mulrow CD, Teutsch SM, et al. Current methods of the US Preventive Services Task Force: A review of the process. Am J Prev Med 2001; 20(3S):21-35.

50.　　GRADE Working Group. Grading quality of evidence and strength of recommendations. Brit Med J 2004; 328(7454):1490.

51.　　Dobscha SK, Campbell R, Morasco BJ, Freeman M, Helfand M. Pain in patients with polytrauma: A systematic review. Washington, DC: Department of Veterans Affairs, 2008. Available at: http://www.hsrd.research.va.gov/publications/esp/Pain-in-Polytrauma-2008.pdf.

52.　　Gaylord KM, Cooper DB, Mercado JM, Kennedy JE, Yoder LH, Holcomb JB. Incidence of posttraumatic stress disorder and mild traumatic brain injury in burned service members: Preliminary report. J Trauma 2008; 64(2S):200-205.

53.　　Ruff RL, Ruff SS, Wang XF. Headaches among Operation Iraqi Freedom/Operation Enduring Freedom veterans with mild traumatic brain injury associated with exposures to explosions. J Rehabil Res Dev 2008; 45(7):941-952.

54.　　Koenigs M, Huey ED, Raymont V, Cheon B, Solomon J, Wassermann EM, et al. Focal brain damage protects against post-traumatic stress disorder in combat veterans. Nat Neurosci 2008; 11(2):232-237.

55.　　Schneiderman AI, Braver ER, Kang HK. Understanding sequelae of injury mechanisms and mild traumatic brain injury incurred during the conflicts in Iraq and Afghanistan: Persistent postconcussive symptoms and posttraumatic stress disorder. Am J Epidemiol 2008; 167(12):1446-1452.

56.　　Schwartz I, Tsenter J, Shochina M, Shiri S, Kedary M, Katz-Leurer M, et al. Rehabilitation outcomes of terror victims with multiple traumas. Arch Phys Med Rehabil 2007; 88(4):440-448.

57.   Bombardier CH, Fann JR, Temkin N, Esselman PC, Pelzer E, Keough M, et al. Posttraumatic stress disorder symptoms during the first six months after traumatic brain injury. J Neuropsych Clin Neurosci 2006; 18(4):501-508.

58.   Greenspan AI, Stringer AY, Phillips VL, Hammond FM, Goldstein FC. Symptoms of post-traumatic stress: Intrusion and avoidance 6 and 12 months after TBI. Brain Inj 2006; 20(7):733-742.

59.   Creamer M, O'Donnell ML, Pattison P. Amnesia, traumatic brain injury, and posttraumatic stress disorder: A methodological inquiry. Behav Res Ther 2005; 43(10):1383-1389.

60.   Gil S, Caspi Y, Ben Ari IZ, Koren D, Klein E. Does memory of a traumatic event increase the risk for posttraumatic stress disorder in patients with traumatic brain injury? A prospective study. Am J Psychiatry 2005; 162(5):963-969.

61.   Jones C, Harvey AG, Brewin CR. Traumatic brain injury, dissociation, and posttraumatic stress disorder in road traffic accident survivors. J Trauma Stress 2005; 18(3):181-191.

62.   Sumpter RE, McMillan TM. Misdiagnosis of post-traumatic stress disorder following severe traumatic brain injury. Br J Psychiatry 2005; 186:423-426.

63.   Ashman TA, Spielman LA, Hibbard MR, Silver JM, Chandna T, Gordon WA. Psychiatric challenges in the first 6 years after traumatic brain injury: Cross-sequential analyses of Axis I disorders. Arch Phys Med Rehabil 2004; 85(4S2):36-42.

64.   Williams WH, Evans JJ, Wilson BA, Needham P. Brief report: Prevalence of post-traumatic stress disorder symptoms after severe traumatic brain injury in a representative community sample. Brain Inj 2002; 16(8):673-679.

65.   Berthier ML, Kulisevsky JJ, Gironell A, Lopez OL. Obsessivecompulsive disorder and traumatic brain injury: Behavioral, cognitive, and neuroimaging findings. Neuropsychiatry Neuropsychol Behav Neurol 2001; 14(1):23-31.

66.   Hoofien D, Gilboa A, Vakil E, Donovick PJ. Traumatic brain injury (TBI) 10-20 years later: A comprehensive outcome study of psychiatric symptomatology, cognitive abilities and psychosocial functioning. Brain Inj 2001; 15(3):189-209.

67.   McCauley SR, Boake C, Levin HS, Contant CF, Song JX. Postconcussional disorder following mild to moderate traumatic brain injury: Anxiety, depression, and social support as risk factors and comorbidities. J Clin Exp Neuropsychol 2001; 23(6):792-808.

68.   Bryant RA, Harvey AG. Postconcussive symptoms and posttraumatic stress disorder after mild traumatic brain injury. J Nerv Ment Dis 1999; 187(5):302-305.

69.   Bryant RA, Harvey AG. The influence of traumatic brain injury on acute stress disorder and post-traumatic stress disorder following motor vehicle accidents. Brain Inj 1999; 13(1):15-22.

70.   Bryant RA, Harvey AG. Relationship between acute stress disorder and posttraumatic stress disorder following mild traumatic brain injury. Am J Psychiatry 1998; 155(5):625-629.

71.   Hibbard MR, Uysal S, Kepler K, Bogdany J, Silver J. Axis I psychopathology in individuals with traumatic brain injury. J Head Trauma Rehabil 1998; 13(4):24-39.

72.   Hickling EJ, Gillen R, Blanchard EB, Buckley T, Taylor A. Traumatic brain injury and posttraumatic stress disorder: A preliminary investigation of neuropsychological test results in PTSD secondary to motor vehicle accidents. Brain Inj 1998; 12(4):265-274.

73.   Trudeau DL, Anderson J, Hansen LM, Shagalov DN, Schmoller J, Nugent S, et al. Findings of mild traumatic brain injury in combat veterans with PTSD and a history of blast concussion. J Neuropsych Clin Neurosci 1998; 10(3):308-313.

74.   Warden DL, Labbate LA, Salazar AM, Nelson R, Sheley E, Staudenmeier J, et al. Post-traumatic stress disorder in patients with traumatic brain injury and amnesia for the event? J Neuropsych Clin Neurosci 1997; 9(1):18-22.

75.   Powell JH, Al Adawi S, Morgan J, Greenwood RJ. Motivational deficits after brain injury: Effects of bromocriptine in 11 patients. J Neurol Neurosurg psychiatry 1996; 60(4):416-421.

76.   Middelboe T, Andersen HS, Birket-Smith M, Friis ML. Minor head injury: Impact on general health after 1 year. A prospective follow-up study. Acta Neurol Scand 1992; 85(1):5-9.

77.   Powell TJ, Collin C, Sutton K. A follow-up study of patients hospitalized after minor head injury. Disabil Rehabil 1996; 18(5):231-237.

78.   Turnbull SJ, Campbell EA, Swann IJ. Post-traumatic stress disorder symptoms following a head injury: Does amnesia for the event influence the development of symptoms? Brain Inj 2001; 15(9):775-785.

79.   Brenner LA, Ladley-O'Brien SE, Harwood JEF, Filley CM, Kelly JP, Homaifar BY et al. An exploratory study of neuroimaging, neurologic, and neuropsychological findings in veterans with traumatic brain injury and/or posttraumatic stress disorder. Mil Med 2009; 174(4):347-352.

80.   Chalton LD, McMillan TM. Can 'partial' PTSD explain differences in diagnosis of PTSD by questionnaire self-report and interview after head injury? Brain Inj 2009; 23(2):77-82.

81.   Mora AG, Ritenour AE, Wade CE, Holcomb JB, Blackbourne LH, Gaylord KM. Post-traumatic stress disorder in combat casualties with burns sustaining primary blast and concussive injuries. J Trauma 2009;66:S178-S185.

82.   Bryant RA, Moulds M, Guthrie R, Nixon RD. Treating acute stress disorder following mild traumatic brain injury. Am J Psychiatry 2003; 160(3):585-587.

83.   Harvey AG, Bryant RA. Acute stress disorder after mild traumatic brain injury. J Nerv Ment Dis 1998; 186(6):333-337.

84.   Batten SV, Pollack SJ. Integrative outpatient treatment for returning service members. J Clin Psychol 2008; 64(8):928-939.

85.   McGrath J. Cognitive impairment associated with post-traumatic stress disorder and minor head injury: A case report. Neuropsych Rehabil 1997; 7(3): 231-239.

86.   Whiting P, Rutjes AW, Reitsma JB, Bossuyt PM, Kleijnen J. The development of QUADAS: A tool for the quality assessment of studies of diagnostic accuracy included in systematic reviews. BMC Med Res Methodol 2003; 3:25.

87.   von Elm E, Altman DG, Egger M, Pocock SJ, Gotzsche PC, Vandenbroucke JP. The Strengthening the Reporting of Observational Studies in Epidemiology (STROBE) statement: Guidelines for reporting observational studies. Ann Intern Med 2007; 147(8):573-577.

88.   Schwartz I, Tuchner M, Tsenter J, Shochina M, Shoshan Y, Katz-Leurer M, Meiner Z. Cognitive and functional outcomes of terror victims who suffered from traumatic brain injury. Brain Inj. 2008; 22(3):255-263.

89.   Bryant RA, Marosszeky JE, Crooks J, Gurka JA. Posttraumatic stress disorder after severe traumatic brain injury. Am J Psychiatry. 2000; 157(4):629-631.

90.   Bryant RA, Marosszeky JE, Crooks J, Baguley I, Gurka J. Coping style and post-traumatic stress disorder following severe traumatic brain injury. Brain Inj. 2000; 14(2):175-180.

91.   Bryant RA, Marosszeky JE, Crooks J, Baguley IJ, Gurka JA. Posttraumatic stress disorder and psychosocial functioning after severe traumatic brain injury. J Nerv Ment Dis. 2001; 189(2):109-113.

92.   Bryant RA, Marosszeky JE, Crooks J, Gurka JA. Elevated resting heart rate as a predictor of posttraumatic stress disorder after severe traumatic brain injury. Psychosom Med. 2004; 66(5):760-761.

93.   Harvey AG, Bryant RA. Two-year prospective evaluation of the relationship between acute stress disorder and posttraumatic stress disorder following mild traumatic brain injury. Am J Psychiatry. 2000; 157(4):626-628.

APPENDIX A: SEARCH STRATEGY

Our study search coordinator, in consultation with our evidence synthesis team, developed the following search strategy. The PubMed and PsycINFO databases were searched for the following terms:

TBI – brain injury (and variants of injury); coma; coma, post-head injury; Glasgow Coma Scale; head injuries, closed; post-concussion syndrome; brain concussion; post-concussive; and brain injury, chronic.

PTSD - combat disorders (and variants of disorder); posttraumatic stress; posttraumatic stress disorder (and variants of disorder); post-traumatic stress disorder (and variants of disorder); stress disorders, post-traumatic; anxiety; and anxiety disorders.

The results from the TBI and PTSD searches were merged attempting to identify studies that included participants with both TBI and PTSD. The search was limited to English language studies of human subjects published between 1980 and 2009.

Sample Search Strategy:

1	brain injur*.mp. or exp Brain Injuries
2	coma.mp. or Coma, Post-Head Injury/ or Coma/ or Glasgow Coma Scale
3	Head Injuries, Closed/ or Post-Concussion Syndrome/ or Brain Concussion/ or post-concussive.mp. or Brain Injury, Chronic
4	combat disord*.mp. or exp Combat Disorders
5	(posttraumatic stress or posttraumatic stress disorder* or post-traumatic stress disorder* or ptsd).mp. or exp Stress Disorders, Post-Traumatic
6	anxiety.mp. or exp Anxiety/ or exp Anxiety Disorders
7	or/1-3
8	or/4-6
9	7 and 8
10	limit 9 to English language
11	limit 10 to yr="1980 - 2009"
12	limit 11 to human

In addition, the REHABDATA database was searched as follows:

From the advanced search page at www.naric.com/research/rehab/advanced.cfm,
Used "All the words" field,
Searched for "brain injuries posttraumatic."
[Provided by Jessica Chaiken of the National Rehabilitation Information Center (NARIC)]

Results of the database searches were combined and duplicate entries eliminated.

APPENDIX B: DATA ABSTRACTION FORM

TBI/PTSD Review
Article Abstraction Form

Author (first):_____

Journal:_____

Year Publication: _____

Country:_____ (where study performed)

Reviewer:_____

VERIFICATION/SELECTION OF STUDY ELIGIBILITY

Article published after 1980	Yes	No	Unclear
English-language	Yes	No	Unclear
Adult Population	Yes	No	Unclear
Subjects with probable TBI	Yes	No	Unclear
Subjects with probable PTSD	Yes	No	Unclear
Report peer-reviewed	Yes	No	Unclear

Other reason for exclusion? (if yes, specify) _____

DESIGN (circle)
Systematic review
Randomized controlled clinical trial
Non-randomized controlled clinical trial
Historical clinical trial
Cohort study
Case-control study
Cross-sectional study
Case series
Case report
Qualitative
Editorial/opinion piece/letter
Undefined

KEY QUESTION(S) (circle)
KQ1: Epidemiology
KQ2: Assessment
KQ3: Treatment
Background

NOTES:
☐ Study contains/may contain same data as another study (specify: _____)
☐ Study described high-quality RCT involving ASD

PARTICIPANTS

Single site or Multi-center?   *(circle one)*   Number of sites _____

Setting: DoD   VAMC   Other   *(circle one)*

Total # of participants   _____

Total # eligible   _____

Reported response rate   _____

Participants excluded from analysis _____ (Why? _____)

	n and %				
	TBI/PTSD	**TBI only**	**PTSD only**	**Neither**	**Total**
# Participants:					
# with PTSD					
# with TBI					
Mild TBI (*How defined?*)					
Moderate TBI (*How defined?*)					
Severe TBI (*How defined?*)					
Age (M, SD)					
Men					
Women					
Race: white					
Race: black					
Race: other					
Ethnicity: Hispanic					
Ethnicity: non-Hispanic					
Active Duty					
Veteran					
Community					

	n and %				
	TBI/PTSD	TBI only	PTSD only	Neither	Total
Education: <HS					
Education: HS grad					
Education: Some college/Associates					
Education: College grad					
Education: Other *(specify)*					
Years of Education (M, SD)					
Service-connected/ disabled					
Seeking SC/ disability					
Trauma: Combat					
Trauma: Terror					
(If combat or terror, specify blast vs. non-blast and any data on distance from blast)					
Trauma: MVC					
Trauma: Assault					
Trauma: Other *(specify)*					
Time since trauma (M, SD) in months					
Number of traumas (M, SD)					
Previous head injury					
Comorbid: Depression					
Comorbid: SUD					
Comorbid: Pain					
Comorbid: Other *(specify)*					

NOTES:

METHODS OF ASSESSMENT

When were assessments made relative to trauma? _____

TBI Assessment	How defined (cut-off score)	n (%)	Gold-standard test; cut-off score	Blinded rater?	Measure of diagnostic accuracy (and statistical uncertainty)
			If measured:		
Self-report (*specify*)					
Clinic screening (*specify: ie, VA screen*)					
Diagnosis (*specify: ie, clinical interview, neuropsych based, etc.*)					
Administrative data					
Other (*specify*)					
PTSD Assessment					
Self-report (*specify*)					
Clinic screening (*specify: ie VA 4-item screen*)					
Diagnosis (*specify: ie, structured interview*)					
Administrative data					
Other (*specify*)					

NOTES:
(i.e., any indication of poorer performance of assessment method when conditions are co-occurring?)

METHODS OF ASSESSMENT

Neuropsych Tests	Check if used:	Notes
Wechsler Adult Intelligence Scale (WAIS-III)		
Stroop Color/Word		
Aphasia Tests (multiple)		
Wechsler Memory Scale – III		
Rey Ostereith Complex Figure		
Wisconsin Card Sorting		
Rey Auditory Verbal Learning Test		
MMPI		
Controlled Oral Word Association (COWA)		
Trail Making Test		
Boston Naming		
Finger Tapping		
Other (specify)		
Other (specify)		
Other (specify)		
Imaging		
EEG		
CT		
MRI		
fMRI		
PET		
SPECT		
Other (specify)		

TREATMENT OUTCOMES   *(use additional pages for each outcome)*

Note additional KQ3 eligibility criteria:			
at least 80% with both TBI/PTSD	Yes	No	Unclear
- or -			
outcome stratified by comorbidity	Yes	No	Unclear

Treatment/intervention(s) of interest:

Outcome of interest and how measured:

	Treatment group 1 *(specify)* *(n =)*	Treatment group 2 *(specify)* *(n =)*	Treatment group 3 *(specify)* *(n =)*	Comparator *(specify)* *(n =)*
Baseline (mean, SD/SE)				
0 - 6 mos. posttreatment (mean, SD/SE)				
6 mos. - 1 year posttreatment (mean, SD/SE)				
1+ year posttreatment (mean, SD/SE)				
Other time frame *(specify)* (mean, SD/SE)				

NOTES:
(i.e., any evidence of adverse events/harms?)

APPENDIX C: PEER REVIEWER COMMENTS

Reviewer Comments	Authors' Responses
1. Are the objectives, scope, and methods for this review clearly described?	
Strengthen review by using "history of TBI" and "sequelae of TBI" or "symptoms associated (or possibly associated) with history of TBI."	Done.
Consider clarifying comorbid and comorbidity – maybe simpler to say that we meant PTSD in those with history of TBI or TBI in those who meet criteria for current PTSD.	We have defined and clarified our use of the terms "TBI," "PTSD," and "comorbidity" in the background section and throughout the revised report.
Use "other mental health conditions and anxiety disorders other than PTSD or anxiety symptoms unspecified" (PTSD is an anxiety disorder so use of terms "mental health comorbidities" and "anxiety" can be confusing at first read).	Changed statements throughout the revised report to read as recommended.
Add more rationale for focus on mTBI given the political context in which it takes place.	We have included a brief additional statement regarding the political importance and rationale for focusing on mTBI.
Explicitly state the reason for including the RAND study given that it is not peer-reviewed and not meeting inclusion criteria. Were other reports rejected?	A statement has been inserted. This study was peer reviewed. Though not published in a peer-reviewed journal, it is published by RAND and readily available on the RAND website. Additional rationale were provided in the draft report indicating that this was one of the largest and most nationally representative studies assessing TBI and PTSD in military personnel who had served in Iraq and Afghanistan. Therefore, it provides key evidence in examining TBI/PTSD prevalence.
We should be clear that this literature search is about people with a history of mTBI who are currently diagnosed with PTSD.	We have attempted to clarify this. Our search was broad. We included any study that assessed reported prevalence of individuals with mTBI and PTSD. Authors frequently referred to these individuals as having "comorbid" TBI and PTSD. However, we agree that the more accurate term for mTBI is "history of…" and have clarified this in our revised report.
Use Hoge review to clarify language – use post-concussive symptoms rather than TBI – for lasting symptoms that result from TBI; consider including paragraph about "language" or "terminology" at the beginning of the review.	We appreciate this suggestion and have been more clear throughout the report in terms of "TBI history," "symptoms related to a TBI," and "comorbidity."
2. Is there any indication of bias in our synthesis of the evidence?	
Inclusion of the RAND report without more justification may give impression of bias (note statement on pg. 30 that RAND report may provide the most reliable estimate …) – consider how study is weighted given that it is not peer reviewed; perhaps findings should be classified as secondary findings?	We have reworded the referenced statement on pg. 30 and provided further rationale for our inclusion of this report. As noted above, the RAND report includes a statement that it underwent peer review with multiple reviewers. The nature of comments and authors' responses to these comments are not available. However, in our experience, the extent of peer review and number of reviewers on evidence reports (as witnessed by this VA ESP report) are typically greater than with most manuscripts submitted for publication in refereed journals. The final report is published on the RAND website. Whether it would have been accepted by a traditional paper journal is not known but we suspect condensed versions would have met journal publication criteria.
Some indication (in introduction) of belief that mTBI is associated with negative outcomes when this is the case in the minority of cases.	We have modified the introduction to include more information on the natural history of mTBI, including evidence that the majority of cases do not have long-term sequelae.

Reviewer Comments	Authors' Responses
No; wondered why CH was a reviewer when he was a contributor with study; probably wanted unbiased reviewer; CH's research is controversial as noted on pg. 2.	Reviewers frequently have a bias. Often our goal is to seek a selection of reviewers that will ensure a broad range of opinions and comments. Prior publication history does not disqualify a reviewer. In general, we select reviewers without disclosure of the names of other reviewers, including the TAP members.
3. Are there any studies on the epidemiology, assessment, or treatment of TBI/PTSD that we may have overlooked?	
Suggest including Bryant study (Ref #33) in Exec. Summary (80% TBI subjects go on to develop PTSD).	The referenced study was included under secondary findings because it did not meet the study inclusion criteria (did not include participants with probable or diagnosed PTSD), which were developed *a priori* in consultation with our TAP. Consistent with previous ESP report formats, we did not include secondary findings in our Executive Summary.
Terrio et al. paper.	The suggested paper did not meet the study inclusion criteria (did not include data on probable or diagnosed PTSD).
Terrio (if PTSD).	We have updated our search through June, 2009. The following additional studies met inclusion criteria and were added to the evidence synthesis review: Brenner et al., 2009; Chalton et al., 2009; and Mora et al., 2009.
4. Additional comments	
Question 1 re comorbid TBI and PTSC is flawed; TBI is acute injury event while PTSD requires symptoms and impairment existing for a defined period of time AFTER the traumatic event; it would be correct to ask how often a TBI injury event may precede the onset of PTSD and whether TBI is a risk factor for PTSD; association may or may not be causal; it also would be correct to ask about comorbidity between PTSD and the sequelae or persistent symptoms/impairment resulting from TBI injury event; need accepted and valid case definition of sequelae attributed to mTBI/concussion; need to examine how strong the evidence is for causal association between mTBI/ concussion and persistent symptoms, sequelae, or impairment (see recent IOM report).	The questions addressed in this evidence synthesis review were developed with considerable input from the VA ESP and specifically our TAP, with the purpose of addressing key questions of clinical and health policy importance and to inform the work of a VA consensus conference on this topic. We agree with the reviewer that the term "comorbid TBI and PTSD" is problematic especially when referring to mTBI. We had discussed the controversy surrounding this issue in our Introduction, Discussion and Future Research Recommendations sections. We have reviewed and further clarified these issues in the revised report. We strongly believe, and included in both our oral presentation at the consensus conference and in this report, that future research is needed to address the issues described by the reviewer.
It is correct to ask about how PTSD may affect, mediate, or confound the expression of symptoms attributed to an mTBI/concussion event (see 2008 NEJM); requires case-definition for dependent variable under study (e.g., symptom sequelae).	We agree and have spoken to this in our Limitations and Future Research Recommendations sections.
Report incorrectly applies the term prevalence; prevalence cannot be determined using the current definitions; technically correct to present the prevalence of PTSD in study participant *who had a history* of TBI (should not use present tense – see Figure 3); never correct to present prevalence of PTSD in those *with* TBI since TBI definition refers to past injury event (see Figure 2); figure should show prevalence of comorbid PTSD and persistent symptoms/sequelae attributed to TBI; lack of clarity by not separating mTBI from moderate and severe TBI for Question 1; inconsistent with Questions 2 and 3.	We have clarified throughout the revised report our intent to examine the prevalence of PTSD in individuals with a history of TBI. Our background clarifies that we addressed TBI with an emphasis on mTBI. For KQ1, we sought to examine prevalence of PTSD in individuals with a history of mTBI versus moderate or severe TBI. As such, our figures denote (when authors provided such information) the prevalence of mTBI history separate from moderate or severe TBI. For KQ2 and KQ3, we sought to assess diagnostic accuracy and treatment effectiveness versus harms for adults specifically with mTBI history who have PTSD.

Reviewer Comments	Authors' Responses
Questions 2 and 3 are flawed for the same reasons; the mTBI/concussion (past injury event) cannot (and should not) be the focus of diagnosis and treatment at time PTSD is diagnosed; questions would only be valid if asked about accuracy or diagnosis and treatment of sequelae of mTBI/concussion in presence of PTSD (with definition of sequelae)	We disagree.
Need consistent and accurate terminology in characterizing the sequelae attributed to concussion/mTBI; "post-concussive symptoms" encompasses the entire spectrum of physical, neurocognitive, and behavioral symptoms attributed to concussion/mTBI; need agreement on the nature of the symptoms – medical, functional somatic syndromes, or related conditions.	We agree and have clarified our wording throughout the report.
Report addresses questions that cannot be answered; questions are ill-conceived; need to first address limitations of current concussion/mTBI definition, derive valid case definition for sequelae attributed to concussion/mTBI, and broaden the focus beyond PTSD.	We agree that future research is needed to address limitations of current case definitions of mTBI. This has been discussed in the report. As noted above, we disagree that the key questions were ill-conceived.
Classification or designation of TBI as an event, diagnosis, sequelae confusing; suggest careful editing, defining of terms, and rephrasing/ reframing of results to address these concerns.	We thank the reviewer and have edited the report to address these concerns.
- EXECUTIVE SUMMARY	
Restate key questions in results section.	We attempted to follow a standard VA ESP report format and have not restated key questions in the results section of the Executive Summary. However, key questions are restated in the Results section of the main report.
8% cut-off for <18 years old unclear – need to state rationale (make change in full report also).	We have edited the report to reflect our 10% cut-off for children <18 years of age.
- INTRODUCTION/BACKGROUND	
Acknowledge that symptoms associated with mTBI in civilian cases generally resolve within weeks to months (1st paragraph of intro gives impression that mTBI is typically associated with negative outcomes).	We have edited this section to include evidence on the natural history of mTBI.
First sentence of 4th paragraph in background is inaccurate ("making an accurate diagnosis …"); think what was meant was "determining etiology of presenting problems in individuals who have a history of TBI and PTSD"; paragraph gives impression that symptoms are needed for TBI diagnosis and that persistent symptoms are common in mTBI (suggest reworking).	We appreciate the reviewer's suggestion and have reworked the referenced paragraph.
Research on usefulness of education for mTBI is limited to education within a relatively short time period post-injury.	We have edited the relevant paragraph to address this comment.
Page 5 second paragraph difficult to follow.	We have clarified this paragraph.
May want to include DoD/VA definition of TBI in addition to CDC definition (Policy Memo October 2007).	Because the operational definitions are similar, we have retained the CDC definition in the report.
Did it matter whether diagnosis of mTBI was first followed by PTSD? Does it matter where initial evaluation starts … mental health or neurology?	We noted in the report that the reported prevalence of TBI/PTSD was highly dependent on the construction of the cohort, method and timing of ascertainment, and definitions of disease/injury. The current literature is insufficient to determine whether timing of event/diagnosis influences outcomes or if there are clinically important differences according to where the initial evaluation starts.

Reviewer Comments	Authors' Responses
Comparison chart (pg 3) – several items are controversial.	Unclear comment. We have included the chart as a direct extraction from a published article that we reference. We believe it is important for the reader to have a full range of information. We have included in the text some background on the controversies surrounding case definitions.
Page 4, nice discussion between screening measures and clinician confirmed diagnosis; also important to mention that VA TBI screening is symptomatic probable TBI (true incidence is difficult to ascertain because positive TBI should be designated as such with or without continued symptoms); VA/DoD report a positive TBI screen as a symptomatic positive patient with probable TBI.	We thank the reviewer and have included a statement about the VA/DOD screening.
- METHODS	
Add special section outlining and addressing some of the issues CH raises.	We have added further information to the Discussion section. Our Future Research Recommendations section had previously discussed these issues.
- RESULTS	
More interested in prevalence of PTSD in a particular group of veterans who have suffered TBI than the overall prevalence of comorbid PTSD and TBI in the overall sample.	We reported the findings according to our key questions where data were available from published evidence. We have included a separate figure presenting data on prevalence of PTSD specifically in veterans with a history of mTBI.
RAND study and additional 5 studies not published? If published, why not included with other studies/manuscripts?	See our comment above regarding our rationale for including the RAND study. There were 31 unique published studies and the RAND report included in the evidence review. The other 5 publications met inclusion criteria but described the same study population as one of the 31 "unique" studies.
Flow diagram (fig 1) – what does "probable TBI/PTSD not included" mean? (clarify or reword).	We have clarified this in the diagram. This meant that individuals with a probable history of TBI and/or probable PTSD (as defined in our Methods section) were not included in the study and thus this study did not meet our evidence report inclusion criteria.
Would like to see table of 28 included studies earlier, including study design, quality rating, and population studied (perhaps grouped by population studied as in Table 2); this would be more helpful than current Table 1.	We placed the table in the appendix consistent with the ESP report template. The quality ratings did not directly apply to these studies and we discussed issues regarding applicability.
Would like to see more description and summarization of the findings from higher quality or more relevant studies rather than limited information including ranges across all studies	We have attempted to do this through our emphasis on the RAND report. Relevant to the military and veteran population, this study was the most population-based as investigators attempted to contact a random sample of military veterans across the United States. Additionally, investigators used detailed, previously-established methods for conducting phone interviews. We disagree that providing ranges across studies is not helpful. These help to show the variation in the literature that may result from studies employing different methods for cohort creation, case ascertainment and timing, and definitions of disease/injury. Therefore it is instructive in establishing future research recommendations.
- ACTIVE RESEARCH	
Did not identify any RCTs rather than state that there are none	We have edited accordingly.
More info on methods for Active Research – How many e-mails (effort to secure responses?); type of response from non-VA investigators; portfolio mgrs other than HSR&D?	A brief statement has been inserted. We acknowledge that our methods likely do not achieve rigorous scientific quality measures. This was an attempt to identify with limited resources high profile active research. The purpose was to guide policy makers, funders, and researchers to ongoing studies and assist in future research planning.

Reviewer Comments	Authors' Responses
- FUTURE RESEARCH	
Add to future research (pg 31) the need to review "systems issues" and coordination with different specialties – there is a real need to figure out ways to get the various specialties together to do treatment planning (Batten & Pollack, 2008 discuss this need).	We appreciate this suggestion and have added this suggestion to our Discussion.
Explicit recommendations that researchers come to a consensus as to measures to be used in this research so that findings can be pooled/compared more easily.	We agree with this suggestion and have clarified this section in our Discussion.
Don't understand ascertainment bias; term "overlapping conditions" is confusing; don't understand 1st sentence of last paragraph (p 31).	We have attempted to clarify these parts of the Discussion section. Ascertainment bias refers to problems with how the cases were defined, identified, and enrolled in a given study that could systematically skew the association(s) under investigation. This could occur because of selection of non-representative study populations, non-representative study participants, timing of the case assessment relative to the injury event, or individuals being aware of the purpose of the assessment and potential gains/harms from a certain response. Each of these alone could potentially result in study outcomes that are biased and not truly reflective of the actual prevalence of TBI/PTSD.
- OVERALL	
Overall, the manuscript is very well written. Thanks for doing this.	We thank the reviewers for their guidance and positive feedback.
I am impressed with this comprehensive report and I found the figures and tables very useful!	Thank you.

APPENDIX D: EVIDENCE TABLES

TABLE 1. Details of published studies evaluated in Key Question 1

Study/ Country	Study design and population	n	Characteristics of participants	Prevalence of TBI history with PTSD	Traumatic brain injury definition/ measure	Post-traumatic stress disorder assessment
Brenner 2009[80] United States	Cross-sectional Veterans receiving services related to TBI and/or PTSD	N=72; 82% (n=59) with TBI; 63% with PTSD (n=45)	*Data for all study subjects* Trauma etiology: NR TBI severity: 46% mild; 17% moderate; 36% severe Time of assessment or since trauma: Median = 23 years (1-53) Mean age: 52 (9.7) years Women: 10% Race: Caucasian 65%; Hispanic 19%; African American 10%; Other 4% Education: Less than high school 3%; high school graduate 26%; more than high school 71% Pain: NR Other mental health conditions: NR	44% (n=32) of all subjects [89% of subjects with mild TBI; 36% of subjects with moderate TBI; 19% of severe TBI]	Interview and chart review.	Structured Clinical Interview for DSM-IV (SCID-IV).
Chalton 2009[81] United Kingdom	Cross-sectional Patients recruited from a hospital outpatient head injury clinic	N=21; all TBI	*Data for all study subjects* Trauma etiology: MVC 43%; fall 29%; assault 24%; work-related accident 5% TBI severity: 19% mild; 19% moderate; 62% severe Time of assessment or since trauma: 3-359 mos (median = 14) Mean age: 42.90 (10.98) Women: 33% Race: NR Education: 12.61 (2.85) years Pain: NR Other mental health conditions: 60% anxious (30% mild; 30% moderate or severe); 35% depressed (15% mild; 15% moderate)	14% (n=3) of all subjects [0% of subjects with mild TBI; 50% of subjects with moderate TBI; 8% of subjects with severe TBI]	Retrospective assessment of post-traumatic amnesia.	Clinician Administered PTSD Scale (CAPS).

Study/ Country	Study design and population	n	Characteristics of participants	Prevalence of TBI history with PTSD	Traumatic brain injury definition/ measure	Post-traumatic stress disorder assessment
Mora 2009[82] United States	Cross-sectional Record review of OEF/OIF soldiers with and without blast injuries treated at the United States Army Institute of Surgical Research Burn Center	n=119 22% with PTSD; 18% with TBI (all but one mTBI)	*Data for all study subjects* Trauma etiology: Military 100% TBI severity: Mild 95%; severe 5% (n=1) Time of assessment or since trauma: 193.7 (171.9) days for blast injury group; 189.7 (175.2) days for no blast injury group Mean age: 26.3 (6.1) for blast injury group; 25.9 (6.0) for no blast injury group Women: 15% blast injury group; 4% no blast injury group Race: NR Education: NR Pain: NR Other mental health conditions: NR	6% (n=7) of all subjects; 35% of mTBI subjects (PTSD status for 1 severe TBI case not reported)	Record review, loss of consciousness served as definition for mTBI.	Self report through PCL-M (> 44 required for PTSD diagnosis).
Gaylord 2008[52] United States	Cross-sectional Service members identified through Trauma Burn Registry	n=76, 31 with TBI	*Data for all study subjects* Burned veterans, TBI vs. no TBI Trauma etiology: Combat (blast and burn) 100% TBI severity: mild 100% Time of assessment or since trauma: NR Mean age: 26 Women: 4% Race: NR Education: NR Pain: NR Other mental health conditions: NR	18% (n=14) of all subjects; 45% of TBI subjects	Medical records and clinical interviews. Glasgow Coma Scale (≥ 13), loss of consciousness (< 30 mins) and/ or post-traumatic amnesia (≤ 24 h).	Self-report through PTSD Checklist (PCL-M). Score of 44+ indicative of PTSD.
Ruff 2008[53] United States	Cross-sectional Subjects evaluated as part of care in VA Medical Center	n=126; all TBI	*Data for all study subjects* OEF/OIF war veterans Trauma etiology: Combat (blast) 100% TBI severity: mild 100% Time of assessment or since trauma: 30 mos (range 8 mos - 4.5 years) Mean age: NR Gender: NR Race: NR Education: NR Pain: 63% (headache) Other mental health conditions: NR	66% (n=83) of all subjects	Administrative data based on positive Veterans Affairs (VA) 4-item TBI screen, including loss of consciousness (< 30 mins) and/ or post-traumatic amnesia (< 24 h) and/or alteration of consciousness (< 24 h).	Self-report through PCL. Score of 50+ indicative of PTSD.

Study/ Country	Study design and population	n	Characteristics of participants	Prevalence of TBI history with PTSD	Traumatic brain injury definition/ measure	Post-traumatic stress disorder assessment
Hoge 2008[22] United States	Cross-sectional Army infantry soldiers surveyed while on duty	n=2525 819 injured; 384 with TBI. 1706 not injured	*Data for all study subjects* Iraq war veterans Trauma etiology (subjects with TBI, can have more than one source of injury): Blast/explosion 75%; fall 29%; MVC 22% TBI severity: mild 100% Time of assessment or since trauma: 3-4 mos post-deployment Mean age: NR Women: 5% Race: NR Education: less than HS 42%; HS grad 58% Pain: 30% (arm, leg, or joint pain; most frequently endorsed pain); 11% (headache) Other mental health conditions: Depression 11%	5% (n=125) of all subjects; 33% of TBI subjects	Self-report, a) loss of consciousness (n=124 subjects); and b) altered mental status (dazed, confused loss of memory) (n=260 subjects).	Self-report through PCL. Score of 50+ indicative of PTSD.
Koenigs 2008[54] United States	Cohort Vietnam veterans in the Vietnam Head Injury Study	n=245; 193 with TBI	*Data for all study subjects* Vietnam veterans Trauma etiology: Combat 100% TBI severity: penetrating 100% Time of assessment or since trauma: NR Mean age: NR Gender: NR Race: NR Education: NR Pain: NR Other mental health conditions: NR	25% (n=62) of all subjects; 32% of TBI subjects	NR.	Structured clinical interview (SCID), based on DSM-IV criteria.
Schneider-man 2008[55] United States	Cross-sectional Surveyed OEF/OIF veterans who served prior to October 2004 and lived in geographic catchment area	n=2235; 275 with TBI	*Data for all study subjects* OEF/OIF war veterans Trauma etiology (could have more than 1): Combat 34% (blast 74%, non-blast 26%); falls 39%; sports/physical training 28%; MVC 20% TBI severity: mild 100% Time of assessment or since trauma: NR Age groups: 18-25 18%; 26-30 15%; 31-35 16%; 36-40 17%; 41+ 38% Women: 13% Race: NR Education: NR Pain: NR Other mental health conditions: NR	5% (n=109) of all subjects; 39% of TBI subjects	Self report, Brief Traumatic Brain Injury Screen.	Self report through PCL. Score of 50+ indicative of PTSD.

57

Study/ Country	n	Study design and population	Characteristics of participants	Prevalence of TBI history with PTSD	Traumatic brain injury definition/ measure	Post-traumatic stress disorder assessment
Schwartz 2007;[57] Schwartz 2008[88] Israel	n=144; 38 with TBI	Case-control, terror vs. non-terror Patients treated in hospital PM&R unit	*Data for all study subjects* Trauma etiology: Terror subgroup - blast 70%, gunshot 30%. Non-terror subgroup – MVC 82%; fall 17% TBI severity: mild 32%; moderate 21%; severe 47% Time of assessment or since trauma: end of rehab stay – terror 218 ± 131days, non-terror 152 ± 114 days Mean age (range): 30 (9-76) Women: 33% Race: NR Education: Less than HS 15%; HS grad 47%; "student" 8%; college grad 29% Pain: NR Other mental health conditions: NR	11% (n=16) of all subjects; 42% of TBI subjects in terror subgroup; 42% of TBI subjects in non-terror subgroup [Prevalence not reported by TBI severity]	Based on Glasgow Coma Scale scores and brain computed tomography (CT).	Semi-structured interview; Revised PTSD Inventory (Solomon et al., 1993). Instrument based on Brief Symptoms Inventory.
Bombardier 2006[58] United States	n=125; all TBI	Cohort Subjects recruited from trauma hospital	*Data for all study subjects* Trauma etiology: MVC 49%; assault 7% TBI severity: mild 44%; moderate 30%, severe 27% Time of assessment or since trauma: NR Mean age: 43 Women: 23% Race: white 92%; black 6% Education: HS grad 85% Pain: NR Other mental health conditions: 71% of TBI/ PTSD subjects had a history of depression or anxiety symptoms unspecified	11% (n=14) of all subjects [9% (n=5) with mild TBI; 8% (n=3) with moderate TBI; 18% (n=6) with severe TBI]	Medical record, based on Glasgow Coma Scale score.	PCL administered as a structured interview. Score of moderate severity on one intrusive, three avoidant, and two arousal symptoms indicative of PTSD.
Greenspan 2006[59] United States	n=198; all TBI	Cohort Subjects identified from TBI databases after discharge from trauma hospitals	*Data for all study subjects* Trauma etiology: MVC 70%; fall 16%, pedestrian injury 6%; other 8% TBI severity: mild 19%; moderate 21%; severe 60% Time of assessment or since trauma: 3 years Mean age: 35 Women: 34% Race: white 74%; black 23%; other 3% Education: Less than HS grad 32%; HS grad 34%; at least some college 34% Pain: NR Other mental health conditions: NR	11% (n=22) of all subjects at 6 mos post-injury; 16% at 12 mos post-injury [Prevalence not reported by TBI severity]	Received treatment for head injury at hospital.	Self-report through the IES. Score of 35+ indicative of PTSD.

Study/ Country	Study design and population	n	Characteristics of participants	Prevalence of TBI history with PTSD	Traumatic brain injury definition/ measure	Post-traumatic stress disorder assessment
Creamer 2005[60] Australia	Cohort Subjects were consecutive admissions to a level 1 trauma hospital	n=307; 189 with TBI	*Data for all study subjects* Trauma etiology: NR TBI severity: mild 100% Time of assessment or since trauma: mean 8 days Mean age: 37 Women: 24% Race: NR Education: NR Pain: NR Other mental health conditions: NR	8% (n=24) of all subjects; 15% of TBI subjects	Loss of consciousness of ≤ 30 minutes, PTA ≤ 24 hours, and GCS of ≥ 13 30 minutes post-trauma.	CAPS, amnesia eliminated as a symptom.
Gil 2005[61] Israel	Cross-sectional Recruited from 2 surgery wards after treatment for TBI	n=120; all TBI	*Data for all study subjects* Trauma etiology: MVC 90% TBI severity: mild 100% Time of assessment or since trauma: within 24 h after hospitalization; 7-10 days, 4 weeks, 6 mos Mean age: 31.4 Women: 42% Race: NR Education: 13 years (mean) Pain: NR Other mental health conditions: NR	14% (n=17) of all subjects at 6 mos post-injury	Presenting to hospital/ clinic for TBI (all had GCS 13-15).	CAPS.
Jones 2005[62] England	Cohort Subjects were consecutive patients in hospital Accident and Emergency Department	n=131; 66 with TBI 118 at 6 weeks; 56 with TBI 74 at 3 mos; 58 with TBI	*Data for all study subjects* Trauma etiology: MVC 100% TBI severity: mild 100% Time of assessment or since trauma: 6 weeks and 3 mos Mean age (range): 37 (18-65) Women: 60% Race: NR Education: NR Pain: NR Other mental health conditions: NR	14% (n=17) of all subjects at 6 weeks; 30% of TBI subjects 14% (n=10) of all subjects at 3 mos; 17% of TBI subjects	Post-traumatic amnesia (< 24 h), as described by Gronwall and Wrightson (1980).	PTSD Symptom Scale (PSS). Amnesia eliminated as a symptom.
Sumpter 2005[63] United Kingdom	Cross-sectional Subjects recruited from community outpatient and rehabilitation services, and volunteer organizations	n=34; all TBI	*Data for all study subjects* Trauma etiology: MVC 47%; fall 32%; assault 18%; sports injury 3% TBI severity: severe 100% Time of assessment or since trauma: 6 year (0.6-34) Mean age (range): 40 (20-60) Women: 12% Race: NR Education: NR Pain: NR Other mental health conditions: NR	3% (n=1) of all subjects	NR. Subjects with severe TBI recruited from community out-patient and rehabilitation services and voluntary organizations.	CAPS, requiring clinical judgment of symptoms being related to trauma. (compared to 3 other methods of assessment.)

Study/Country	Study design and population	n	Characteristics of participants	Prevalence of TBI history with PTSD	Traumatic brain injury definition/measure	Post-traumatic stress disorder assessment
Ashman 2004[64] United States	Cohort. Subjects recruited from medical centers, brain injury associations, newspaper and website advertisements, and word-of-mouth	n=188; all TBI. 83 at 24 mos; all TBI	Data for all study subjects. Trauma etiology: NR. TBI severity: mild 29%; moderate-severe 62%; 9% unknown. Time of initial assessment or since trauma: 3mos - 4 years. Mean age (range): 40 (18-87). Women: 47%. Race: white 72%; black 12%. Education: Less than high school 27%; HS/some college 38%; college graduate 25%. Pain: NR. Other mental health conditions at time 1: Depression 35%; Anxiety symptoms unspecified 27%; Substance use disorder (SUD) 14%	30% (n=56) of all subjects at time 1 (initial assessment between 3 mos and 4 years post-injury). 18% (n=34) of all subjects at time 2 (12 mos after initial assessment). 21% (n=17) of all subjects at time 3 (24 mos after initial assessment). [Prevalence not reported by TBI severity]	Self-reported; severity determined using ACRM loss of consciousness criteria.	SCID, based on DSM-IV criteria.
Williams 2002[65] United Kingdom	Cross-sectional. Subjects recruited through brain injury services	n=66; all TBI	Data for all study subjects. Trauma etiology: MVC 45%; falls 18%; assault 3%. TBI severity: severe 100%. Time of assessment or since trauma: mean 5.9 years (range 1-26 years). Mean age (range): 38 (17-70). Women: 24%. Race: NR. Education: mean 12 years (range 9-19 years). Pain: NR. Other mental health conditions: NR	18% (n=12) of all subjects	Self-report, based on loss of consciousness (+6 hrs) and/or post-traumatic amnesia (≥1 day).	Self-report through IES, corroborated by relative or caregiver. Score of 26+ indicative of PTSD.
Berthier 2001[66] Spain	Case series. Consecutive referrals to Behavioral Neurology Unit of a single University Hospital; all patients diagnosed with OCD after TBI	n=10; all TBI (all OCD)	Data for all study subjects. Trauma etiology: MVC 100%. TBI severity: mild 60%; moderate 20%; severe 20%. Time of assessment or since trauma: > 51 mos. Mean age: 30. Women: 60%. Race: NR. Education: mean 11 years. Previous head injury: 0%. Pain: NR. Other mental health conditions: Obsessive-compulsive disorder 100%; depression 90%	70% (n=7) of all subjects [60% (n=6) with mild TBI; 10% (n=1) with moderate TBI; 0% with severe TBI]	Glasgow Coma Scale score, determined at hospital admission.	SCID, based on DSM-III-R criteria.

Study/ Country	n	Study design and population	Characteristics of participants	Prevalence of TBI history with PTSD	Traumatic brain injury definition/ measure	Post-traumatic stress disorder assessment
Hooften 2001[67] Israel	n=76; all TBI	Cohort Participants from a larger longitudinal study of patients from a single neuropsych rehab center with medically documented TBI at least 5 years before study	Data for all study subjects Trauma etiology: MVC 64%; combat 25%; work-related 9% TBI severity: severe 100% Time of assessment or since trauma: 14± 5.8 (SD) years Mean age (range): 25 (17-50) age at injury Women: 83% Race: NR Education: NR Pain: NR Other mental health conditions: Depression 45%	10% (n=7) of 68 responding to PTSD items	Subjects were in a coma for an unspecified long period of time.	Post-Traumatic Stress Disorder Inventory, based on DSM-III criteria. "Probable PTSD" diagnosis assigned to subjects meeting 4 criteria: traumatic event, re-experiencing, numbing, and hyperarousal symptoms.
McCauley 2001[68] United States	n=200; 115 with TBI	Cohort Participants recruited from Emergency Center or inpatient unit of a single Level-1 trauma center	Data for all study subjects Trauma etiology: MVC 69%; assault 15%; other 16% TBI severity: mild 83%; moderate 17% Time of assessment or since trauma: 88 days Mean age: 34 Women: 78% Race: Hispanic 52%; black 32%; white 16% Education: mean 11 years Pain: NR Other mental health conditions: Depression 9%	8% (n=15) of all subjects; 13% of TBI subjects [12% (n=11) of subjects with mild TBI; 15% (n=4) of subjects with moderate TBI]	Hospital admission logs ("non-penetrating head injury" based on Glasgow Coma Scale scores 9-15).	SCID, based on DSM-IV criteria.
Turnball 2001[79] United Kingdom	n=53; all TBI	Cross-sectional Subjects attended an Accident and Emergency Unit following a traumatic event and had evidence of TBI in medical record	Data for all study subjects Trauma etiology: assault 58%; MVC 30%; fall 11% TBI severity: mild 58%; moderate 21%; severe 17%; none 2 subjects Time of assessment or since trauma: 5 mos Mean age: 35 Women: 13% Race: NR Education: NR Pain: NR Other mental health conditions: NR	17-27% of all subjects [Prevalence not reported by TBI severity]	Based on history of post-traumatic amnesia.	Those with IES-R score ≥ 20 administered the CAPS, with amnesia excluded as a symptom. Results reported using the most strict and most lenient cutoffs as recommended by scale authors on the CAPS.

Study/Country	Study design and population	n	Characteristics of participants	Prevalence of TBI history with PTSD	Traumatic brain injury definition/measure	Post-traumatic stress disorder assessment
Bryant 1999a,[69] Bryant 2000,[89] Bryant 2000,[90] Bryant 2001,[91] Bryant 2004[92] Australia	Cohort Consecutive admissions to single site major brain injury rehab unit	n=96; all TBI	*Data for all study subjects* Trauma etiology: MVC 73%; industrial injury 15%; assault 13% TBI severity: mild 100% Time since trauma: 6 mos Mean age: 34 Women: 20% Race: NR Education: NR Pain: 58% report daily pain; M = 6.90 (2.65) on a 1-10 severity scale Other mental health conditions: NR	27% (n=26) of all subjects	Medical records based on Glasgow Coma Scale score and post-traumatic amnesia (Westmead PTA scale).	Post-traumatic Stress Disorder Interview (PTSD-I; Watson et al, 1991), based on DSM-III-R criteria.
Bryant 1999b,[70] Australia	Cohort Consecutive admissions to single site major trauma hospital following MVC	n=105; 46 with TBI	*Data for all study subjects* Trauma etiology: MVC 100% TBI severity: mild 100% Time of assessment or since trauma: 6 mos Mean age: 31 Women: 40% Race: NR Education: NR Pain: Headaches in 100% of subjects with mTBI/PTSD Other mental health conditions: NR	9% (n=9) of all subjects; 20% (n=9) of TBI subjects	Hospital admissions, post-traumatic amnesia < 24 h, loss of consciousness.	Composite International Diagnostic Interview (CIDI).
Bryant 1998[71] Harvey 2000[93] Australia	Cohort Consecutive MVC victims treated at a single site major trauma hospital with evidence of TBI	n=79; all TBI	*Data for all study subjects* Trauma etiology: MVC 100% TBI severity: mild 100% Time of assessment or since trauma: mean 7.15 days (range 2-28); PTSD assessed 6 mos and 2 years post-trauma Mean age (range): 29 (16-60) Women: 30% Race: NR Education: NR Pain: NR Other mental health conditions: NR	24% (n=15) of 63 subjects assessed at 6 mos; 22% (n=11) of 50 subjects assessed at 2 years	Hospital admission, post-traumatic amnesia < 24 h.	Composite International Diagnostic Interview (CIDI).

Study/ Country	Study design and population	n	Characteristics of participants	Prevalence of TBI history with PTSD	Traumatic brain injury definition/ measure	Post-traumatic stress disorder assessment
Hibbard 1998[72] United States	Cross-sectional Participants randomly selected from 431 individuals with TBI involved in a larger quality of life survey	n=100; all TBI	*Data for all study subjects* Trauma etiology: MVC 62%; assault 8%; other 30% TBI severity: NR Time of assessment or since trauma: mean 7.6 years Mean age: 40 Women: 47% Race: white 73%; black 14%; Hispanic 9% Education: HS grad or less 29%; some college/ college grad 49% Pain: NR Other mental health conditions: Depression 61%; SUD 28%; obsessive-compulsive disorder (OCD) 15%; panic disorder 14%; phobias 10%; general anxiety disorder 9%	19% (n=19) of all subjects	Self-reported loss of consciousness.	SCID, based on DSM-IV criteria.
Hickling 1998[73] United States	Cross-sectional Subjects were recently in and sought medical treatment within 2 days for MVC	n=107; 16 with TBI	*Data for all study subjects* Trauma etiology: MVC 100% TBI severity: NR Time since trauma: 1-4 mos Mean age: 35.9 Women: 69% Race: 9.3% "minorities" Education: NR Pain: NR Other mental health conditions: NR	8% (n=9) of all subjects; 56% of subjects with TBI (9 of 16)	Clinical screening – rates of TBI stratified across multiple types of injury that varied in likelihood of producing TBI – only strictest criterion (e.g., loss of consciousness) used in the present review as evidence of TBI.	Clinician-Administered PTSD Scale (CAPS).
Trudeau 1998[74] United States	Cross-sectional Outpatient male combat veterans from a PTSD treatment program and/ or addictive disorders treatment program with a diagnosis of PTSD	n=43; all PTSD	*Data for all study subjects* Trauma etiology: Combat 100% *(27 with a blast concussion and 16 without)* TBI severity: mild 60%; moderate 40% Time of assessment or since trauma: NR Mean age (range): 52 (26-72) Women: 0% Race: NR Education: NR Pain: NR Other mental health conditions: SUD 42%; Attention-deficit/hyperactivity disorder (ADHD) 16%	60% (n=25) of 42 respondents [Prevalence not reported by TBI severity]	Self-report, either a) being in the presence at a detonation of ordnance, often resulting in death or serious injury to others closer to blast, b) experiencing unconsciousness for ≤ 20 mins or dazed for ≥ 1 hour without loss of consciousness, or c) requiring medical attention for concussive episode.	Not described, all subjects were enrolled in a PTSD recovery program and/or addictive disorders treatment program and had a clinical diagnosis of PTSD.

Study/ Country	Study design and population	n	Characteristics of participants	Prevalence of TBI history with PTSD	Traumatic brain injury definition/ measure	Post-traumatic stress disorder assessment
Warden 1997[75] United States	Cohort Consecutive active duty service members with a moderate TBI at Walter Reed Army Medical Center	n=41; all TBI	*Data for all study subjects* Trauma etiology: MVC 70%; fall 19%; assault 9% TBI severity: moderate 100% Time of assessment or since trauma: 4-29 mos Mean age: 27 Women: 2% Race: NR Education: NR Pain: NR Other mental health conditions: NR	11% (n=3) of 28 subjects at 8 weeks post-injury; 20% (n=3) of 15 subjects at 6 mos post-injury; n=0 of 18 subjects at 12 mos post-injury; 14% (n=1) of 7 subjects at 24 mos post-injury	Based on history of post-traumatic amnesia and Rancho Los Amigos scale.	Present State Examination, additional PTSD questions added to assess full spectrum of PTSD symptoms (e.g., added symptoms about re-experiencing and avoidance). Memory of event not required. Administered by clinicians.
Powell 1996[76] United Kingdom	Cohort Participants recruited from a hospital who were admitted for observation following mild/ moderate TBI	n=35; all TBI	*Data for all study subjects* Trauma etiology: MVC 34%; dom. assault 29%; assault 14%; sport/other 14%; industrial 3% TBI severity: mild 69%; moderate 31% Time of assessment or since trauma: 3 mos Mean age: 35 Women: 34% Race: NR Education: NR Pain: NR Other mental health conditions: Depression 9%	34% (n=12) of all subjects [25% of subjects with mild TBI; 55% of subjects with moderate TBI]	Based on Glasgow Coma Scale, subjects admitted to hospital for minor head injury.	Self report through IES (>26 required for a positive screen for PTSD).
Sbordone 1995[21] United States	Cross-sectional Participants diagnosed with post-concussive syndrome or PTSD prior to study recruitment; No information provided on method or location of recruitment	n=70; 28 with TBI, 42 with PTSD	*Data for all study subjects* Trauma etiology: MVC 66%; blunt head trauma 14%; fall 10%; other 10% TBI severity: mild 100% Time of assessment or since trauma: TBI 20.8 ± 16.4 mos; PTSD 29.1 ± 32.7 mos Mean age: 37 Women: 41% Race: NR Education: NR Pain: NR Other mental health conditions: NR	0 TBI subjects had PTSD	Unstructured interview by first author.	Unstructured interview by first author.

Study/ Country	Study design and population	n	Characteristics of participants	Prevalence of TBI history with PTSD	Traumatic brain injury definition/ measure	Post-traumatic stress disorder assessment
Middelboe 1992[77]

Denmark | Cohort

Consecutive patients admitted to a hospital Neurology Department with clinical evidence of TBI | n=28; all TBI | *Data for all study subjects* Trauma etiology: NR TBI severity: mild 100% Time since trauma: 3 mos & 1 year Mean age: 37 Women: 46% Race: NR Education: NR Pain: 32% reported headaches at 1 year post-TBI Other mental health conditions: NR | 0 subjects had PTSD; 11% with "high" IES scores (above 19) 1 year post-trauma | Through neurologic exam (not specified). | Self-report through IES and unspecified symptom checklist. Information regarding how PTSD diagnosis was established not provided. |

TABLE 2. Details of RAND study evaluated in Key Question 1

Study/ Country	Study design and population	n	Characteristics of participants	Prevalence of TBI history with PTSD	Traumatic brain injury definition/ measure	Post-traumatic stress disorder assessment
RAND 2008[5] United States	Cross-sectional OEF/OIF service members and veterans identified through random digit dialing using telephone exchanges encompassing 24 geographic areas	n=1965; 19.5% with TBI (weighted percentage)	*Data for all study subjects* Trauma etiology: Military 100% TBI severity: NR Time of assessment or since trauma: NR. Time since deployment was 35% 0-17 mos, 33% 18-35 mos, 33% 36 mos or greater Median age: 30 Women: 12% Race: white 66%; non-white 34% Education: NR Pain: NR Other mental health conditions: Probable major depression 14%	6.6% of all subjects; 34% of TBI subjects (weighted percentages)	Self report, Brief Traumatic Brain Injury Screen.	Self report through PCL-M.

APPENDIX E: ACTIVE RESEARCH FINDINGS

TABLE 1. Ongoing research: Epidemiology of TBI/PTSD (Key Question #1)

Principal Investigator	Project Title/Status	Main Objective(s)	Study Characteristics
Copeland, L.	Tracking OEF/OIF Transition from DoD to VA Status: Completed, article in preparation	1. Determine feasibility of DoD-to-VA transfer of PHI on a local level 2. Determine rate of transition of Wounded Warriors from Brooke Army Medical Center to VA healthcare system 3. Determine use of VA mental healthcare NOTE: TBI diagnosis obtained from medical records	Study Design: Observational cohort Population: OEF/OIF deployed personnel treated and discharged from Brooke Army Medical Center (BAMC) FY02-FY07 Intervention: None Comparator: None Outcomes: Prevalence of PTSD at BAMC and at VA; delay from discharge at DoD to diagnosis/treatment of PTSD in VA system Timing: From discharge at DoD to treatment at VA Setting: Army Medical Center and VA sites
Donnelly, K. (See Appendix E, Table 2)	Cognitive Assessment of Veterans after Traumatic Brain Injury Status: In progress	1. Describe war-related cognitive and affective symptoms and patterns of substance abuse in OEF/OIF veterans 2. Construct cognitive and affective profiles of OEF/OIF veterans over time 3. Describe the temporal relationship between composite stress index and cognitive profiles of OEF/OIF veterans 4. Describe the temporal relationships among TBI, cognitive symptoms, patient outcomes, and health services outcomes	Study Design: Prospective cohort Population: 500 OEF/OIF veterans Intervention: None Comparator: None Outcomes: TBI identified with structured diagnostic interview; PTSD identified with PTSD checklist Timing: Baseline, 6, 12, and 18 mos Setting: 5 outpatient VA sites (VISN 2)
Griffin, J.	Understanding and Meeting the Needs of Informal Caregivers to Improve Outcomes for TBI patients with Polytrauma Status: In progress	Assess the relationship between caregiving and patient, caregiver, and family health outcomes, including the physical, emotional, and financial burden of caregiving and the resources available to caregivers	Study Design: Observational Population: Family caregivers of all OEF/OIF patients with a TBI discharged from a Polytrauma Rehabilitation Center (PRC) Intervention: None Comparator: None Outcomes: Caregiver-report of patients' TBI and PTSD diagnoses Timing: At least 3 mos post-discharge from PRC Setting: Surveys administered by mail

Principal Investigator	Project Title/Status	Main Objective(s)	Study Characteristics
Kang, H. (See Appendix E, Table 2)	National Health Study for a New Generation of U.S. Veterans Status: In progress	1. Determine if the health status of OEF/OIF veterans is better, worse, or the same as non-deployed veterans 2. Characterize healthcare utilization and VA disability compensation patterns of OEF/OIF veterans 3. Describe the natural histories of psychological disorders, mTBI, musculoskeletal problems, and other health conditions over time among veterans 4. Obtain prevalence figures for mTBI and PTSD from a population-based sample	Study Design: Longitudinal Population: 30,000 deployed OEF/OIF veterans and 30,000 non-deployed OEF/OIF era veterans Intervention: None Comparator: None Outcomes: TBI and PTSD identified with screening instruments used in VAMCs Timing: 10 year follow-up with assessment every 3 years Setting: Surveys administered by mail, on-line, and by telephone
Polusny, M.	Mild TBI/PTSD Comorbidity and Post-Deployment Outcomes in National Guard Soldiers Status: Completed, manuscripts in preparation	1. Describe the scope of mTBI/PTSD among returning National Guard OIF veterans 2. Identify the extent to which these problems impacted veterans' psychosocial functioning, physical health, and quality of life over time 3. Examine variation in new OIF veterans' experiences with VA by mTBI and probable PTSD status	Study Design: Two-wave longitudinal cohort Population: OIF National Guard soldiers Intervention: None Comparator: None Outcomes assessed: *In-theater:* blast exposure, mTBI, PTSD symptoms; *Post-deployment:* combat exposure, exposure to explosive blasts and injuries sustained, mTBI and post-concussive symptoms, current psychosocial functioning, physical health, access and use of VA healthcare services Timing: In-theater screening one-month before returning home; mailed survey at 1 year post-deployment Setting: In-theater and home
Rao, V.	Post-Traumatic Brain Injury Depression Status: In progress	To identify risk factors for depression among patients with first time TBI (all severity levels) (NOTE: PTSD assessed with full structured interview)	Study Design: Prospective, observational Population: 140 consecutive TBI patients; recruited soon after injury Intervention: None Comparator: None Outcomes: Major depression; also assessing PTSD Timing: Follow-up at 1 year post-injury Setting: Clinical (2 university-affiliated trauma units)
Tupler, L. (See Appendix E, Table 2)	TBI Severity and Associated Neurocognitive findings in OEF/OIF Veterans Status: Data collection complete; analysis in progress	To examine the epidemiology of TBI in OEF/OIF veterans and the relationship between self-reported severity of TBI and level of PTSD symptomatology and neurocognitive performance (NOTE: results to be analyzed by severity of TBI)	Study Design: Prospective, observational Population: Approximately 850 OEF/OIF veterans; TBI and PTSD status unknown by investigators at time of enrollment Intervention: None Comparator: None Outcomes: Neurocognitive and psychological test battery (including PTSD Checklist) findings examined in relation to TBI history (chart review or self-report) Timing: Post-deployment; time from TBI assessed Setting: One Polytrauma Rehabilitation Center, three Level III Polytrauma Support Clinic Teams

TABLE 2. Ongoing research: Assessment of mTBI/PTSD (Key Question #2)

Principal Investigator	Project Title/Status	Main Objective(s)	Study Characteristics
Donnelly, K. (See Appendix E, Table 1)	Cognitive Assessment of Veterans after Traumatic Brain Injury Status: In progress	Describe the psychometric properties of the VA TBI screening tool	Study Design: Prospective cohort Population: 500 OEF/OIF veterans Intervention: None Comparator: None Outcomes: Item analysis of the VA TBI screening tool; test-retest reliability and sensitivity/specificity with structured diagnostic interview for TBI probability/severity as criterion Timing: Baseline, 6, 12, and 18 mos Setting: 5 outpatient VA sites (VISN 2)
Kang, H. (See Appendix E, Table 1)	Markers for the Identification, Norming, and Differentiation of TBI and PTSD (MIND) Status: Planning stage	1. Clarify differential diagnoses between TBI and PTSD 2. Build objective, consistent, and operator-independent diagnostic criteria	Study Design: Cross-sectional Population: Subset of OEF/OIF veterans from New Generation study with TBI and/or PTSD and a comparison group Intervention: None Comparator: None Outcomes: Advanced diagnostic tests (neuroimaging, sleep studies, neuroendocrine measures) Timing: One-time testing; patients continue enrollment in New Generation study Setting: VA War Related Illness and Injury Study Centers
Rao, S. Levin, H.	Neural and Behavioral Sequelae of Blast-Related Traumatic Brain Injury Status: In progress	Identify the similarities and potential differences in the neural and behavioral sequelae of blast-related TBI compared to mechanically-induced TBI occurring in civilians	Study Design: Prospective, cross-sectional observational Population: n=120 in 4 groups – military with mild to moderate TBI, military with mild to moderate orthopedic injury (OI), civilian with mTBI, civilian with OI Intervention: None Comparator: None Outcomes: Advanced MRI findings, neuropsychological test results, post-concussion symptoms, PTSD symptoms, depression, pain and fatigue scales Timing: Assessment at 12-24 mos post-injury Setting: Cleveland and Houston VAMCs; community hospital trauma/rehabilitation centers

Traumatic Brain Injury and Post-Traumatic Stress Disorder

Principal Investigator	Project Title/Status	Main Objective(s)	Study Characteristics
Tupler, L. (See Appendix E, Table 1)	TBI Severity and Associated Neurocognitive findings in OEF/OIF Veterans Status: Data collection complete; analysis in progress	Examine the relationship between self-reported severity of TBI and level of PTSD symptomatology and neurocognitive performance on a measure of premorbid intellectual functioning and prefrontal verbal abstraction (NOTE: results to be analyzed by severity of TBI)	Study Design: Prospective, observational Population: Approximately 850 OEF/OIF veterans; TBI and PTSD status unknown by investigators at time of enrollment Intervention: None Comparator: None Outcomes: Neurocognitive and psychological test battery (including PTSD checklist) findings examined in relation to TBI history (chart review or self-report) Timing: Post-deployment Setting: One Polytrauma Rehabilitation Center, three Level III Polytrauma Support Clinic Teams
Tupler, L.	Posttraumatic Stress Disorder with and without Traumatic Brain Injury: Comorbidity and Longitudinal Course of Recovery Status: Preparing for data analysis	Examine neurocognition in OEF/OIF post-deployed and active-duty personnel with TBI alone, PTSD alone, and comorbid TBI and PTSD compared with combat controls and non-combat controls (NOTE: same population as in study described below)	Study Design: Prospective, observational Population: Approximately 170 OEF/OIF veterans and active-duty personnel Intervention: None Comparator: None Outcomes: Neurocognitive and psychological test battery (including PTSD checklist) findings examined in relation to TBI history (chart review or self-report) Timing: Continuous recruitment since 2006 Setting: One Polytrauma Rehabilitation Center, two Level III Polytrauma Support Clinic Teams
Tupler, L.	Can Olfaction be used to Discriminate Traumatic Brain Injury from Posttraumatic Stress Disorder? Status: Preparing for data analysis	Examine the utility of the University of Pennsylvania Smell Test (UPSIT) as a means of discriminating TBI from PTSD (NOTE: same population as in study described above)	Study Design: Prospective, observational Population: Approximately 170 OEF/OIF veterans and active-duty personnel Intervention: None Comparator: None Outcomes: UPSIT and PTSD Checklist in relation to TBI history (chart review or self report) Timing: Continuous recruitment since 2006 Setting: One Polytrauma Rehabilitation Center, two Level III Polytrauma Support Clinic Teams
Vanderploeg, R. Fitzgerald, S.	TBI Screening Instruments and Processes for Clinical Follow-up Status: In progress	Evaluate the reliability and validity of the existing Traumatic Brain Injury (TBI) Clinical Reminder Screen for OEF/OIF Veterans controlling for comorbidities and demographics	Study Design: Diagnostic test evaluation Population: OEF/OIF veterans Intervention: None Comparator: None Outcomes: Reliability and validity Timing: Not stated Setting: VA Polytrauma Rehabilitation Centers, Network Sites, and Support Clinic Teams

TABLE 3. Ongoing research: Treatment of mTBI/PTSD (Key Question #3)

Principal Investigator	Project Title/Status	Main Objective(s)	Study Characteristics
Beckham, J.	Rehabilitation Strategies to Reduce Violence and Anger in TBI and PTSD Status: Proposal under review	1. Identify risk and protective factors empirically related to violent behavior among veterans who have returned from Iraq and Afghanistan 2. Examine the link between specific factors related to violence among veterans from previous conflicts and post-deployment violence risk among Iraq and Afghanistan veterans 3. Develop an evidence-based risk assessment instrument to administer to Iraq and Afghanistan veterans in order to identify those most in need of services	Study Design: Prospective cohort Population: 300 OEF/OIF veterans and a member of their family Intervention: None Comparator: None Outcomes: Modality of psychotherapy, dosages and classes of psychiatric medications Timing: Interview at baseline and 6 mos Setting: VA, outpatient NOTE: although the direct aim of the study is not to evaluate particular rehabilitation strategies, the investigators believe that information yielded from the study may be useful in sequencing treatment efforts
Epstein, D.	Pilot Test of Preference-Based Insomnia Treatment for OEF/OIF Veterans Status: Proposal under review	Pilot test a brief, preference-based insomnia intervention augmented by audio files (MP3) and web-based resources	Study Design: One group, pre-post Population: 26 OEF/OIF veterans, history of blast exposure or other injury resulting in period of altered consciousness AND insomnia complaint of ≥ 1 mo. duration with daytime impairment, Insomnia Severity Index (ISI) ≥ 10, phone and internet access, ability to listen to audio files on MP3 player Intervention: Multi-component – relaxation therapy, mindfulness exercise, stimulus control instructions, sleep restriction therapy, and sleep education and hygiene Comparator: None Outcomes: ISI, Pittsburgh Sleep Quality Index-Addendum for PTSD (PSQI-A), daily sleep diary, treatment feasibility Timing: 4 week treatment phase, assessed pre-treatment, during treatment, and 2 weeks post-treatment Setting: VA, outpatient
Nichols, L. Martindale-Adams, J.	Team Based Initiative: Support (Pilot) Status: Completed, report in development	1. Determine the feasibility of implementing volunteer support teams with TBI families 2. Identify the obstacles and opportunities in implementation	Study Design: Case series Population: Family members of 6 Guard/Reserve service members (OEF/OIF veterans) with mild-complicated TBI and co-occurring PTSD Intervention: Project coach for needs assessment, team formation, training Comparator: None Outcomes: Qualitative data on family issues and concerns Timing: Returning to community post-injury Setting: Outpatient (family homes), rural

71

Principal Investigator	Project Title/Status	Main Objective(s)	Study Characteristics
Harch, P.	Pilot Study of Hyperbaric Oxygen Therapy (HBOT) in Chronic Traumatic Brain Injury (TBI)/Post-Concussion Syndrome (PCS) and TBI/Post-Traumatic Stress Disorder (PTSD) Status: In progress	Determine if one or two 40-treatment courses of low pressure HBOT can improve cognition and brain imaging in subjects with either chronic mild-moderate TBI (also known as PCS), or chronic TBI with PTSD secondary to blast injury	Study Design: Open-label, single group Population: 30 patients (15 with TBI, 16 with TBI and PTSD), 18-45 years old, blast-induced injury resulting in mTBI/concussion with loss of consciousness; able to manage self-care Intervention: 40 (or 80) HBOT sessions; 2 sessions per day for 20 days (4 weeks) Comparator: None Outcomes: Psychometric and neuropsychological tests, brain imaging Timing: Injury 1 to 4 years prior to enrollment baseline assessment, post-treatment assessment, and follow-up at 6 mos and 1 year post-treatment Setting: Non-VA clinic
Ruff, R.	Improving Sleep: Initial Treatment in OIF/OEF Veterans with Blast-Induced Mild TBI Status: Completed, publication in development	Determine if treating impaired sleep would reduce headache frequency and severity	Study Design: Case series Population: OIF/OEF veterans with headaches associated with mTBI and persisting neurocognitive deficits Intervention: Education in sleep hygiene and prazosin to reduce nightmares associated with PTSD Comparator: Patients who do not complete prazosin protocol or who discontinued prazosin after intervention period Outcomes: Headache frequency and severity, cognitive assessment, sleep assessment Timing: Assessment at baseline, after 9 week intervention, 6 mo. follow-up Setting: Outpatients from VAMC

www.ingramcontent.com/pod-product-compliance
Lightning Source LLC
Chambersburg PA
CBHW081600170526
45166CB00009B/2763